ICD-10-PCS Coder Training Manual 2011

Prepared by the
Professional Practice Resources Team
American Health Information
Management Association

Contributing Authors
Ann Barta, MSA, RHIA
*Kathryn DeVault, RHIA, CCS, CCS-P wrote test
Ann Zeisset, RHIT, CCS, CCS-P

Contributors
Melanie Endicott, MBA/HCM, RHIA, CCS, CCS-P
Anita Majerowicz, MS, RHIA

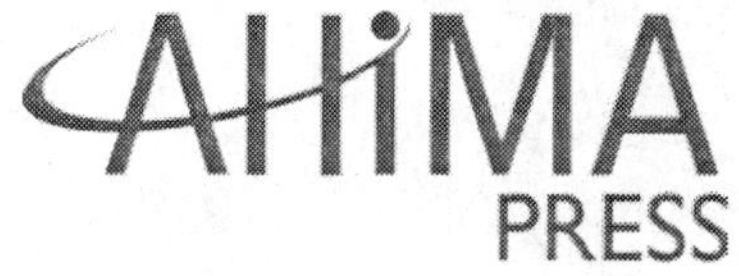

AHIMA Product No.: AC207811
ISBN: 978-1-58426-288-6

AHIMA Staff:
Katie Greenock, Editorial and Production Coordinator
Ashley Sullivan, Assistant Editor
Pamela Woolf, Senior Developmental Editor
Ken Zielske, Director of Publications

American Health Information Management Association
233 North Michigan Avenue, 21st Floor
Chicago, Illinois 60601-5809
www.ahima.org

Contents

About the Authors

Ann Barta, MSA, RHIA, Professional Practice Resources Specialist, provides professional expertise on ICD-10 issues to AHIMA members, the media, and outside organizations. She is responsible for the development and presentation of educational materials on ICD-10-CM/PCS. In addition, she authors materials for and supports AHIMA online coding education, publications, and other products as they relate to ICD-10-CM/PCS. Ms. Barta also serves as faculty for the AHIMA ICD-10-CM/PCS Academies.

Prior to joining AHIMA in September 2008, Ms. Barta participated in a one-year contract between the AHIMA Foundation of Research and Education and Centers for Medicare and Medicaid Services (CMS) to determine potential impacts to CMS when converting from ICD-9-CM to ICD-10-CM/PCS coding systems. Prior to that, Ms. Barta served as a corporate coding manager for a large healthcare system. She has more than 30 years experience as an HIM director and coding consultant. She has been an educator of coding and HIM for more than 15 years, served as an Associate Dean for Health Sciences, and was system coordinator for an RHIT program.

As an AHIMA member, Ms. Barta participated in various leadership positions. She has served on various RHIT Program Advisory Boards. Additionally, she was actively involved with the Illinois Health Information Management Association, serving on the Education Committee and as a state coding instructor with the implementation of ICD-9-CM. Ms. Barta received her master of science in Health Services Administration from Central Michigan University in Mt. Pleasant, MI.

Kathryn DeVault, RHIA, CCS, CCS-P, is a Professional Practice Resources Manager for AHIMA. In her role, she provides professional expertise to AHIMA members, the media, and outside organizations on professional practice issues. In addition, she authors materials for and supports AHIMA online coding education, including the AHIMA Coding Basics program. Ms. DeVault also serves as a technical advisor for the association on ICD-9-CM, ICD-10, and CPT coding publications. Ms. DeVault also serves as faculty for the AHIMA ICD-10-CM/PCS Academies.

Prior to joining AHIMA in 2008, Ms. DeVault served as data quality analyst for coding in a regional healthcare system. For the past seven years, she has been a coding educator at a local community college. Ms. DeVault has authored many articles and has presented numerous seminars and educational sessions on coding and HIM-related topics.

As an AHIMA member, Ms. DeVault has participated in numerous leadership roles at both the state and regional level through the Colorado Health Information Management Association. She received her bachelor's degree in Liberal Arts from the University of Colorado.

Ann Zeisset, RHIT, CCS, CCS-P, is Manager of Professional Practice Resources for AHIMA. In her role, Ms. Zeisset provides professional expertise to AHIMA members, the media, and outside organizations on coding practice issues. She also authors and supports AHIMA online coding education, including the Coding Basics program and is a technical advisor for the association on ICD-9-CM, CPT, and ICD-10-CM/PCS coding publications. Ms. Zeisset has also authored several publications.

Prior to joining AHIMA in 1999, Ms. Zeisset served as director of Health Information/Utilization Management. Before that, Ms. Zeisset served in various coding roles, and has been an educator of coding and HIM for more than 20 years at multiple colleges, and currently serves as adjunct faculty in the Health Information Management Program at the University of Cincinnati. Ms. Zeisset has authored many coding related articles and has presented numerous seminars and educational sessions on coding and other HIM-related topics throughout the United States including many for home health professionals.

Ms. Zeisset recently completed a one-year contract between the Foundation for Research and Education and CMS to determine potential impacts to CMS when converting from ICD-9-CM to ICD-10-CM/PCS coding systems. Ms. Zeisset is a frequent author and speaker on ICD-10-CM/PCS and serves as faculty for the AHIMA ICD-10-CM/PCS Academies.

Ms. Zeisset was awarded the Distinguished Member award from SILHIMA in 2003, the Certified Coding Specialist award in 2005, and the Professional Achievement award from ILHIMA in 2010. Ms. Zeisset received a bachelor's degree in Organizational Leadership at Greenville College.

Acknowledgments

The exercises in this book were created using several AHIMA resources as a base. All of the adapted materials underwent a vigorous review to bring them into alignment with the latest versions of the ICD-10-PCS code sets and guidelines which were available at the time of publication.

The author team adapted many of the application exercises in this book from case scenarios originally created by Anita Hazelwood, MLS, RHIA, FAHIMA and Carol Venable, MPH, RAHIA, FAHIMA. The authors also would like to thank Sue Bowman for her contribution to the content and review of this publication. In addition, the authors would like to thank June Bronnert, RHIA, CCS, CCS-P for her contributions.

Preface to the Training Manual

On January 16, 2009, the US Department of Health and Human Services (HHS) published a Final Rule for the adoption of ICD-10-CM and ICD-10-PCS code sets to replace the 30-year-old ICD-9-CM code sets under rules, 45 CFR Parts 160 and 162 of the Health Insurance Portability and Accountability Act of 1996 (HIPAA). The compliance date for the two classification sets was established as October 1, 2013. A second rule related to the HIPAA transaction standards—X12 version 5010 and NCPDP version D.0—establishes earlier effective dates. The HIPAA transactions software must be updated to accommodate the use of the ICD-10-CM and ICD-10-PCS code sets by January 1, 2012 with the exception of Medicaid Pharmacy Subrogation Transactions, which have an effective date of January 1, 2013.

To read the final rules published in the *Federal Register*, please go to the following web sites:

- Modifications to the Health Insurance Portability and Accountability Act (HIPAA) Electronic Transaction Standards (http://edocket.access.gpo.gov/2009/pdf/E9-740.pdf)
- HIPAA Administrative Simplification: Modifications to Medical Data Code Set Standards To Adopt ICD–10–CM and ICD–10–PCS (http://edocket.access.gpo.gov/2009/pdf/E9-743.pdf)

The adoption of ICD-10-CM (diagnoses) will affect all components of the healthcare industry. However, the adoption of ICD-10-PCS will affect only those components of the healthcare industry that currently utilize ICD-9-CM Volume 3—inpatient procedures. Therefore, CPT® and HCPCS Level II will continue to be used for reporting physician and other professional services in addition to procedures performed in hospital outpatient departments and other outpatient facilities.

The three key issues HHS believes necessitate the need to update from ICD-9-CM to ICD-10-CM and ICD-10-PCS are:

- ICD-9-CM is out of date and running out of space for new codes.
- ICD-10 is the international standard to report and monitor diseases and mortality, making it important for the United States to adopt ICD-10-based classifications for reporting and surveillance.
- ICD codes are core elements of many health information technology (HIT) systems, making the conversion to ICD-10-CM/PCS necessary to fully realize benefits of HIT adoption.

The use of ICD-10-CM will offer greater detail and granularity and will greatly enhance HHS's capability to measure quality outcomes, such as the quality performance outcome measures used in the hospital pay-for-reporting program. The greater detail and granularity of ICD-10-CM/PCS will also provide more precision for claims-based, value-based purchased initiatives such as the hospital-acquired condition (HAC) payment policy.

In addition, the transition to ICD-10-CM/PCS will ultimately facilitate realizing the benefits of using interoperability standards specified by the Healthcare

Information Technology Standards Panel (HITSP), including SNOMED-CT®. The benefits of using SNOMED-CT increase if such use is linked to classification systems such as ICD-10-CM and ICD-10-PCS. Mapping would be used to link SNOMED-CT to these new code sets, and plans are underway to develop these maps.

How to Use This Manual

The AHIMA Academy for ICD-10-PCS Trainers is primarily designed to prepare individuals to train others in ICD-10-PCS through course content that focuses on instruction in the code set. The *ICD-10-PCS Coder Training Manual 2011* is designed to be used by students who are trained by AHIMA Academy ICD-10-PCS trainers to build upon their basic knowledge of ICD-10-PCS fundamentals. Although the implementation date for ICD-10-CM/PCS is several years away, it is necessary that individuals responsible for training are fully knowledgeable of the code sets in order to prepare students and the workforce for the transition. Transitioning curriculum from ICD-9-CM to ICD-10-CM/PCS will present unique challenges for academicians. Educating the workforce will also require that the healthcare industry begin planning and preparing for the new code sets.

The content of the *ICD-10-PCS Coder Training Manual 2011* is based on the January 2011 release of the *International Classification of Diseases, Tenth Revision, Procedure Coding System (ICD-10-PCS)*, which can be downloaded from the following web site: http://www.cms.hhs.gov/ICD10

The *ICD-10-PCS Coder Training Manual 2011* contains many references to and explanations of ICD-10-PCS coding guidelines and conventions. It includes ICD-10-PCS coding exercises at the basic, intermediate, and advanced level. These coding exercises emphasize all aspects of the coding classification system so students can apply their knowledge of coding principles and definitions. Answers to the coding exercises are provided.

Students should recognize that additional, self-directed study will be required to master the guidelines and principles of ICD-10-PCS coding beyond the materials provided in this manual. In addition, many students will require additional coursework to increase their level of knowledge in anatomy, physiology, pathophysiology, pharmacology, and medical terminology. Because ICD-10-PCS requires a stronger background in the biomedical sciences, instructors should develop plans for assessing their students' strengths/weaknesses in these areas. Identifying students' learning needs and levels of knowledge is crucial to preparing a solid educational transition plan.

In addition to this text, students of the AHIMA Academy will use the 2011 *ICD-10-PCS: The Complete Official Draft Code Set* code book (Ingenix) to complete the practice exercises.

Introduction: ICD-10-PCS Overview

Section 1 – ICD-10-PCS History, Structure, and Organization

History of ICD-10-PCS and General Structure

Introduction to ICD-10-PCS

Since 1979, the reporting of procedures for hospital inpatients has been done using Volume 3 of the *International Classification of Diseases, Ninth Revision, Clinical Modification* (ICD-9-CM). This system is highly outdated and incapable of further expansion to identify specific levels of detail to classify procedure codes. In 1992, the Centers for Medicare & Medicaid Services (CMS) funded the project to develop the *International Classification of Diseases, Tenth Revision, Procedure Classification System* (ICD-10-PCS) with 3M Health Information Systems. ICD-10-PCS will be implemented in the United States on October 1, 2013, to capture hospital inpatient procedure codes. ICD-10-PCS has a multiaxial seven-character alphanumeric code structure providing unique codes for procedures. ICD-10-PCS currently undergoes annual updates.

There were four key attributes that were considered during the development of ICD-10-PCS. The following table defines these characteristics.

Key Attributes of ICD-10-PCS

Attribute	**Definition**
Completeness	A unique code for each substantially different procedure
Expandability	Structure should allow easy expansion
Multiaxial	Should contain independent characters and an individual axis that maintains its meaning across ranges of codes
Standardized Terminology	Definitions are well defined, with no multiple meanings, and each term is assigned a specific meaning

Note: Meeting these objectives should allow coders to construct accurate codes with minimal effort.

In the development of ICD-10-PCS, several general principles were followed:

- *Diagnostic Information is Not Included in Procedure Description* – When procedures are performed for specific diseases or disorders, the disease or disorder is not contained in the procedure code. There are no codes for procedures exclusive to aneurysms, cleft lip, strictures, neoplasms, hernias, etc. The diagnosis codes, not the procedure codes, specify the disease or disorder.
- *Not Otherwise Specified (NOS) Options are Restricted* – ICD-9-CM often provides a "not otherwise specified" code option. Certain NOS options made available in ICD-10-PCS are restricted to the uses laid out in the ICD-10-PCS draft guidelines. A minimal level of specificity is required for each component of the procedure.
- *Limited Use of "Not Elsewhere Classified" (NEC) Option* – ICD-9-CM often provides a "not elsewhere classified" code option. Because all significant components of a procedure are specified in ICD-10-PCS, there is generally no need for an NEC code option. However, limited NEC options are incorporated into the classification system where necessary. For example, new devices are frequently developed, and therefore it is necessary to provide an "Other Device" option for use until the new device can be explicitly added to the coding system.
- *Level of Specificity* – All procedures currently performed can be specified in ICD-10-PCS. The frequency with which a procedure is performed was not a consideration in the development of the system. Rather, a unique code is available for variations of a procedure that can be performed.

Source: CMS 2011a

ICD-10-PCS Code Structure

One of the reasons ICD-10-PCS was created was because there were structural problems with ICD-9-CM. In addition, specific objectives, essential characteristics, and general guidelines were established for the development of a procedural coding system in order to meet today's coded data requirements. Therefore, one would expect the structure of ICD-10-PCS to be quite different than ICD-9-CM Volume 3.

With the ICD-10 implementation, the US clinical modification of the ICD will not include a procedure classification based on the same principles of organization as the diagnosis classification. Instead, a separate procedure coding system has been developed to meet the rigorous and varied demands that are made of coded data in the healthcare industry. This represents a significant step toward building a health information infrastructure that functions optimally in the electronic age.

The following table provides a comparison between the structure of ICD-9-CM and ICD-10-PCS.

ICD-9-CM Volume 3	ICD-10-PCS
Follows ICD structure (designed for diagnosis coding)	Designed and developed to meet healthcare needs for a procedure coding system
Codes available as fixed/finite set in list form	Codes constructed from flexible code components (values) using Tables
Codes are 3–4 digits long with a decimal point placed after the second digit	Codes are seven characters long
Codes are numeric	Codes are alphanumeric

Source: CMS 2011b

The following is a table from the CMS 2011 Development of the ICD-10 Procedure Coding System (ICD-10-PCS), which provides a comparison of ICD-9-CM and ICD-10-PCS using the NCVHS (National Committee on Vital and Health Statistics) characteristics.

NCVHS Characteristics	ICD-9-CM	ICD-10-PCS
Hierarchical Structure: Ability to aggregate data from individual codes into larger categories	**Hierarchical Structure:** The ability to aggregate by body system is provided but there is no ability to aggregate by other components of a procedure	**Hierarchical Structure:** The ability to aggregate across all essential components of a procedure is provided
Each code has a unique definition forever—not reused	Some codes do not have a unique definition because the codes have been reused	All codes have a unique definition

Expandability: Flexibility to new procedures and technologies ("empty" code numbers) Mechanism for periodic updating Code expansion must not disrupt systematic code structure	**Expandability:** Minimal flexibility. New procedures and technologies are difficult to incorporate. Virtually no empty code numbers. Updated annually through Coordination and Maintenance Committee Code expansions are difficult to incorporate without disrupting systematic code structure	**Expandability:** Extensive flexibility. New procedures and technologies are easily incorporated. Unlimited empty code values available. Update process needs to be established. If ICD-10-PCS replaces ICD-9-CM, Coordination and Maintenance Committee would be responsible for update process. Code expansions do not disrupt systematic structure.
Comprehensive: Provides NOS and NEC categories so that all possible procedures can be classified somewhere Includes all types of procedures Applicability to all settings and types of providers	**Comprehensive:** Extensive use of NOS and NEC categories. All procedures can be categorized somewhere. Broad NOS and NEC categories result in procedure codes which are ambiguously defined. All types of procedures are included although there is minimal detail for many types of procedures. All settings and types of providers are covered, although there is minimal detail for many settings and types of providers.	**Comprehensive:** Limited use of NOS and NEC categories. NEC and NOS categories are specific to each axis of code. All procedures can be categorized somewhere. Procedure codes are precisely defined even when NOS and NEC options are used. All types of procedures are included except evaluation and management procedures. Complete detail is provided for all types of procedures All settings and types of providers are covered except physician office services for evaluation and management. Complete detail is provided for all settings and types of providers.

Non-Overlapping: Each procedure (or component of a procedure) is assigned to only one code.	**Non-Overlapping:** The same procedure when performed for different diagnoses is sometimes assigned to multiple codes.	**Non-Overlapping:** Each procedure is assigned to only one code.
Ease of Use: Standardization of definitions and terminology Adequate indexing and annotation for all users	**Ease of Use:** No standard definitions provided. Terminology is inconsistent across codes. Full index but specificity of index varies across codes	**Ease of Use:** All terminology is precisely defined. All terminology is used constantly across all codes. Full index. Index is computer-generated so specificity of index is consistent across codes.
Setting and Provider Neutrality: Same code regardless of who or where procedure is performed	**Setting and Provider Neutrality:** Codes are independent of who or where procedure is performed	**Setting and Provider Neutrality:** Codes are independent of who or where procedure is performed
Multiaxial: Body system(s) affected Technology used Techniques/approaches used Physiological effect or pharmacological properties Characteristics/composition of implant	**Multiaxial:** Body system affected can be determined from code number Limited and inconsistent specification of technology used Limited and inconsistent specification of techniques/ approaches used Limited and inconsistent specification of physiological effect and pharmacological properties Limited and inconsistent specification of characteristics/ composition of implant	**Multiaxial:** A specific character in the code specifies the body system affected Technology used is specified in the approach character of the code Techniques/approaches used are specific in the approach character of the code Physiological effect and pharmacological properties are specified when relevant to the procedure Characteristics/composition of implants are specified in the device character of the code

Limited to Classification of Procedures: Should not include diagnostic information Other data elements (such as age) should be elsewhere in the records	Limited to Classification of Procedures: Diagnostic information is included in some codes No other data elements included in code	Limited to Classification of Procedures: No diagnostic information is included in the code No other data elements included in code

Source: CMS 2011a

The process of constructing codes in ICD-10-PCS is logical and consistent: individual letters and numbers, referred to as "values," are selected in sequence to occupy the seven spaces of the code, referred to as "characters."

All codes in ICD-10-PCS are seven characters in length and each of the seven characters represent an aspect of the procedure. The following diagram illustrates the seven characters of a code from the main section of ICD-10-PCS, the Medical and Surgical section.

Character 1 Section	Character 2 Body System	Character 3 Root Operation	Character 4 Body Part	Character 5 Approach	Character 6 Device	Character 7 Qualifier

One of 34 values can be assigned to each character in an ICD-10-PCS code; the numbers 0 through 9 and the alphabet (except [the letters] I and O) are utilized. I and O are not used to eliminate the possible confusion with the numbers 1 and 0. An example of an ICD-10-PCS code is: 0T9B70Z. This code was constructed by choosing a specific value for each of the seven characters. Based on details about the procedure performed, values for each character specifying the section, body system, root operation, body part, approach, device and qualifier are assigned.

Due to the fact that the definition of each character of the code is a function of its physical position in the code, the same value placed in a different position in the code has a different meaning. For example, the value 0 in the first character means something different than the value 0 in the second character.

Next the code 0LB50ZZ, "Excision of right lower arm and wrist tendon, open" will be utilized to illustrate the meanings of each of the seven characters of a code from the Medical and Surgical section of ICD-10-PCS.

The first character of a code determines the broad procedure category, or section, where the code is located. In this example, the section is the Medical and Surgical with "0" representing Medical and Surgical section in the first character.

The second character defines the body system which is the general physiological system or anatomical region involved. Examples of body systems include *central nervous system, upper arteries, respiratory system, tendons, muscles and upper joints.* In this example, the body system is *tendons*, represented by the value of L for the second character.

The third character defines the root operation, or the objective of the procedure being performed. Examples of root operations are *excision, bypass, division and fragmentation.* For this example the root operation is *excision* which has the character value of B.

The fourth character defines the body part or specific anatomical site where the procedure was performed. The body system, second character, provides only a general indication of the procedure site and the body part, fourth character, indicates the precise body part. When the second character is L, the value 5 as the fourth character represents the *right lower arm and wrist tendon.*

The fifth character defines the approach, or the technique used to reach the operative site. Seven different approach values are used in the Medical and Surgical section of ICD-10-PCS. In this example, the approach is *open* and is represented by the value 0.

The sixth character defines the device and depending on the procedure performed, there may or may not be a device left in place at the end of the procedure. Device values fall into four basic categories:

- Grafts and Prostheses
- Implants
- Simple or Mechanical Appliances
- Electronic Appliances

In this example, there is no device left at the operative site, therefore, the value Z is used to represent *no device.*

The seventh character defines a qualifier for a particular code. A qualifier specifies an additional attribute of the procedure, if applicable. In this example, there is no specific qualifier applicable to the procedure, so the value is Z, *no qualifier.*

Character 1 Section	Character 2 Body System	Character 3 Root Operation	Character 4 Body Part	Character 5 Approach	Character 6 Device	Character 7 Qualifier
Medical and Surgical	Tendons	Excision	Lower Arm and Wrist, Right	Open	No Device	No Qualifier
0	**L**	**B**	**5**	**0**	**Z**	**Z**

Source: CMS 2011b

Overall Organization

General Organization

ICD-10-PCS is composed of 16 sections, represented by the numbers 0 through 9 and the letters B through D and F through H. The broad procedure categories contained in these sections range from surgical procedures to substance abuse treatment. The 16 sections are subdivided into three main sections: Medical and Surgical section, Medical and Surgical-related sections and Ancillary sections.

The first section, Medical and Surgical section, contains the majority of procedures typically reported in an inpatient setting. As mentioned previously, all procedure codes in this section begin with the section value of 0. The following diagram illustrates the seven characters of a code from the Medical and Surgical section.

Character 1 Section	Character 2 Body System	Character 3 Root Operation	Character 4 Body Part	Character 5 Approach	Character 6 Device	Character 7 Qualifier

Sections 1 through 9 of ICD-10-PCS comprise the Medical and Surgical-related sections. These sections include the following:

Section Value	**Description**
1	Obstetrics
2	Placement
3	Administration
4	Measurement and Monitoring
5	Extracorporeal Assistance and Performance
6	Extracorporeal Therapies
7	Osteopathic
8	Other Procedures
9	Chiropractic

In sections 1 and 2, all seven characters have the same definition or meaning as the procedures in the Medical and Surgical section.

Codes in sections 3 through 9 are structured for the most part like their counterparts in the Medical and Surgical section, with a few exceptions. For example, in sections 5 and 6, the fifth character is defined as the duration instead of approach.

Additional differences include these uses of the sixth character:

- Section 3 defines the sixth character as substance
- Sections 4 and 5 define the sixth character as function
- Sections 7 through 9 define the sixth character as method

Sections B through D and F through H comprise the Ancillary sections of ICD-10-PCS which includes the following sections:

Section Value	Description
B	Imaging
C	Nuclear Medicine
D	Radiation Oncology
F	Physical Rehabilitation and Diagnostic Audiology
G	Mental Health
H	Substance Abuse Treatment

The definitions of some characters in the Ancillary sections also differ from those seen in the previous sections. For example, in the Imaging section, the third character is defined as the root type, and the fifth and sixth characters define contrast and contrast/qualifier respectively.

Additional differences include:

- Section C defines the fifth character as radionuclide
- Section D defines the fifth character as modality qualifier and the sixth character as isotope
- Section F defines the fifth character as type qualifier and the sixth character as equipment
- Section G and H define the third character as a type qualifier

Source: CMS 2011b

Components of ICD-10-PCS and Table Organization

So far you have learned that the overall organization of the codes within ICD-10-PCS is by section. The next step is to understand how the codes are incorporated into ICD-10-PCS.

There are three components to ICD-10-PCS: the Tables, the Index, and the List of Codes. The ICD-10-PCS Index can be used to access the root operation tables and consists of alphabetized main terms that represent either a root operation value or a common procedure term. The root operation tables provide the valid choices of values available to construct a code. The tables consist of four columns and a varying number of rows with each row specifying the valid choices for the characters 4 through 7. The final component is the list of codes.

Coding Tip: The values for characters 1 through 3 are located at the top of each table. The Index often only provides the first 3-4 characters of the code with the first three characters indicating the correct table to reference.

Note: Contrary to ICD-9-CM, after a coding professional is acquainted with the table structure, it is no longer necessary to first consult the Index when coding in ICD-10-PCS.

Tables – The tables are organized in a series, beginning with section 0, Medical and Surgical, and body system 0, Central Nervous, and proceeding in numerical order. Sections 0 through 9 are followed by sections B through D and F through H. The same convention is followed within each table for the second through the seventh character, numeric values in order first, followed by alphabetical values in order.

The root operation tables consist of four columns and a varying number of rows. Following is an example of the table for the root operation Bypass, in the Central Nervous body system.

0: Medical and Surgical (Section) 0: Central Nervous (Body System) 1: Bypass: Altering the route of passage of the contents of a tubular body part (Root Operation)			
Body Part Character 4	Approach Character 5	Device Character 6	Qualifier Character 7
6 Cerebral Ventricle	0 Open	7 Autologous Tissue Substitute J Synthetic Substitute K Nonautologous Tissue Substitute	0 Nasopharynx 1 Mastoid Sinus 2 Atrium 3 Blood Vessel 4 Pleural Cavity 5 Intestine 6 Peritoneal Cavity 7 Urinary Tract 8 Bone Marrow B Cerebral Cisterns
U Spinal Canal	0 Open	7 Autologous Tissue Substitute J Synthetic Substitute K Nonautologous Tissue Substitute	4 Pleural Cavity 6 Peritoneal Cavity 7 Urinary Tract 9 Fallopian Tube

The values of characters 1 through 3 are provided at the top of each table. Four columns contain the applicable values for characters 4 through 7.

A table may be separated into rows to specify the valid choices of values for characters 4 through 7. In order to build a valid ICD-10-PCS code, the values for characters 4 through 7 must come from the same row. An ICD-10-PCS code built with values from more than one row is considered to be an invalid code.

Index – The ICD-10-PCS Index can be used to access the Tables. The Index mirrors the structure of the Tables, so it follows a consistent pattern of organization and use of hierarchies. The Index is organized as an alphabetic lookup with two types of main terms:

- Based on the value of the third character
- Common procedure terms

For the Medical and Surgical and related sections, the root operation values are used as main terms in the Index. In other sections, the values representing the general type of procedure performed, such as nuclear medicine or imaging type, are listed as main terms.

For the Medical and Surgical and related sections, values such as Bypass, Division, Excision and Transplantation are included as main terms. The applicable body systems or body parts are listed beneath the main term, and refer to a specific table. For the Ancillary sections, values such as Fluoroscopy and Positron Emission Tomography are listed as main terms.

The second type of main terms in the Index are common procedure terms, such as "appendectomy," "colonoscopy," or "hysterectomy." These entries are listed as main term and generally refer to a table or tables from which a valid code can be constructed. For example, the following appears under the main term Cholecystectomy in the Index:

Cholecystectomy

- *see* Excision, Gallbladder 0FB4
- *see* Resection, Gallbladder 0FT4

List of Codes – The ICD-10-PCS List of Codes is a resource which displays all valid codes in alphanumeric order. Each entry begins with the seven character code followed by the full text code description. The code descriptions are generated using rules that produce standardized, complete and easy-to-read code descriptions.

Source: CMS 2011b

Index and Table Conventions

ICD-10-PCS utilizes a number of Index and Table conventions. Following is a summary of selected conventions:

- All codes are seven characters long.
- The definition of each character is a function of its physical position in the code.
- The Tables are organized beginning with the numeric values in order first followed by the alphabetic values in order. For the second through the seventh character value, this same convention is followed within each Table.
- Root Operation Tables contain values for characters 1–3 and four columns providing the valid combinations of values for characters 4–7 required for code creation.
- Each column in the Table may have a varying number of rows. However, a combination of characters not in a single row of a Table is not a valid code.
- Main terms are based on the second and third-character value.
- The root operation values, character 3, are included as main terms for the Medical and Surgical and related sections. For other sections, the general type of procedure performed is listed as a main term.
- Common procedure terms such as appendectomy are also listed as main terms in the Index.

Activity 1: Matching Procedures with Sections

Match the following procedures with the section of ICD-10-PCS where it is found:

1. 8E0H30Z, Acupuncture

2. F07L0ZZ, Manual physical therapy for range of motion and mobility, patient right hip, no special equipment

3. 3E1M39Z, Peritoneal dialysis via indwelling catheter

4. 4A02XM4, Cardiac stress test, single measurement

5. BW03ZZZ, Chest x-ray, AP/PA and lateral views

Section 1 Review Questions

1. Which of the following codes is located in the Medical and Surgical-related sections of ICD-10-PCS?
   a. B342ZZZ
   b. C23GQZZ
   c. HZ94ZZZ
   d. 5A2204Z

2. True or False? ICD-10-PCS has four components.
   a. True
   b. False

3. Complete the following sentence. The third character for codes located in the Medical and Surgical section defines the ____________.
   a. Root Operation
   b. Section
   c. Body System
   d. Body Part

4. Which government agency was responsible for funding the development of ICD-10-PCS?
   a. CDC
   b. NCHS
   c. CMS
   d. NCVHS

Section 2 – ICD-10-PCS Attributes, Characteristics, and Definitions

Key Attributes of ICD-10-PCS

Based on the information covered in Section 1, you now know that ICD-10-PCS is quite different in structure and organization than ICD-9-CM Volume 3. In Section 2, further explanation is provided on the structural attributes of ICD-10-PCS. The three key attributes described—multiaxial structure, completeness, and expandability—were among those that the National Committee on Vital and Health Statistics recommended for a new procedural coding system.

Multiaxial Structure – The key attribute that provides the framework for all other structural attributes is multiaxial code structure. This attribute makes it possible for the ICD-10-PCS to be complete, expandable and to provide a high degree of flexibility and functionality.

ICD-10-PCS codes are composed of seven characters with each character representing a category of information that can be specific about the procedure performed. A character defines both the category of information and its physical position in the code.

A character's position can be understood as a semi-independent axis of classification that allows different specific values to be inserted into the space, and whose physical position remains stable. Within a defined code range, a character retains the general meaning that it confers on any value in that position. For example, the fifth character retains the general meaning "approach" in sections 0 through 4 and 7 through 9.

Each group of values for a character contains all the valid choices in relation to the other characters of the code, giving the system completeness. Additionally, each group of values for a character can be added to as needed, giving the system expandability. Finally, each group of values is confined to its own character, giving ICD-10-PCS a stable, predictable readability across a wide range of codes. ICD-10-PCS' multiaxial structure houses its capacity for completeness, expandability and flexibility, giving it a high degree of functionality for multiple uses.

Completeness – Completeness is considered a key structural attribute for a new procedural coding system. The specific recommendations for completeness include the following characteristics:

- A unique code is available for each significantly different procedure
- Each code retains its unique definition; codes are not reused

In ICD-10-PCS, a unique code can be constructed for every significantly different procedure. Within each section of ICD-10-PCS, a character defines a consistent component of a code, and contains all applicable values for that character. The values define individual expressions (i.e., open, percutaneous) of the character's general meaning (approach) that are then used to construct unique procedure codes. Therefore, all approaches by which a procedure is performed are assigned a separate approach value in the system resulting in every procedure which uses a different approach having its own unique code.

This is true of the other characters of ICD-10-PCS as well. For example, the same procedure performed on a different body part has its own unique code and the same procedure performed using a different device also has its own unique code.

Because ICD-10-PCS codes are constructed of individual values, the unique, stable definition of a code in the system is retained. New values may be added to ICD-10-PCS to represent a specific new approach, device or qualifier, but whole codes by design cannot be given new meaning and reused.

Expandability – Expandability is another key structural attribute of ICD-10-PCS. The specific recommendation for expandability includes the following characteristics:

- Accommodate new procedures and technologies
- Add new codes without disrupting the existing structure

ICD-10-PCS has been designed to be easily updated as new codes are required for new procedures and techniques. All changes to this classification system can be made within the existing structure, because whole codes are not added. Instead, one of the two possible changes is made:

- A new value for a character is added as needed to the classification system
- An existing value for a character is added to a table(s) in the classification system

Source: CMS 2011b

Design Characteristics of ICD-10-PCS

Besides the three key attributes implemented into ICD-10-PCS, there were several additional design characteristics recommended by the National Committee on Vital and Health Statistics and others. As you familiarize yourself with these characteristics, keep in mind how many of the problems identified with ICD-9-CM Volume 3 have been addressed in ICD-10-PCS.

ICD-10-PCS also possesses several additional characteristics in response to government and industry recommendations as follows:

- Standardized terminology within the coding system
- Standardized level of specificity
- No diagnostic information
- No explicit "not otherwise specified" (NOS) code options
- Limited use of "not elsewhere classified" (NEC) code options

Standardized Terminology – Words commonly used in clinical vocabularies may have multiple meanings resulting in confusion and inaccurate data. ICD-10-PCS is standardized and self-contained with characters and values used in the system having specific definitions.

For example, the word "excision" is used to describe a wide variety of surgical procedures. In ICD-10-PCS, the word "excision" describes a single, precise surgical objective, defined as "cutting out or off, without replacement, a portion of a body part."

The terminology used in ICD-10-PCS is standardized to provide precise and stable definitions for all ICD-10-PCS code descriptions. As a result, ICD-10-PCS code descriptions do not include eponyms or common procedure names. This is not the case with ICD-9-CM. For example, ICD-9-CM code descriptor for 22.61 is "excision of lesion of maxillary sinus with Caldwell-Luc approach" and the code descriptor for 51.10 is "endoscopic retrograde cholangiopancreatography." In these two examples the code descriptor refers to either a physician's name or common terms. In ICD-10-PCS physician's names, common terms, and acronyms are not included in a code description. Instead, such procedures are coded to the root operation that accurately identifies the objective of the procedure.

With rare exception, ICD-10-PCS does not define multiple procedures with one code which allows preserving standardized terminology and consistency across the classification system. Therefore, a procedure that meets the reporting criteria for a separate procedure is coded separately in ICD-10-PCS allowing the system to respond to changes in technology and medical practice with the maximum degree of stability and flexibility. This is not the case with ICD-9-CM where we often see procedures that are typically performed together coded with a combination code such as 28.3, "tonsillectomy with adenoidectomy."

Standard Level of Specificity – In ICD-9-CM one procedure code with its description and includes notes often encompasses multiple procedure variations while another code defines a single specific procedure. In contrast, ICD-10-PCS provides a standardized level of specificity for each code, with each code representing a single procedure variation.

In ICD-9-CM code 39.31, "suture of an artery," does not specify the artery, whereas the code range 38.40–38.49, "resection of artery with replacement," specifies the artery by anatomical region at the fourth-digit level of the code. In ICD-10-PCS, the codes identifying all artery suture and artery replacement procedures have the same degree of specificity.

In general, ICD-10-PCS code descriptions are more specific than their ICD-9-CM counterparts, but occasionally an ICD-10-PCS code description is actually less specific. In most instances this is because the ICD-9-CM code contains diagnostic information. ICD-10-PCS uses a standardized level of code specificity which cannot always take into account the fluctuations in the ICD-9-CM level of specificity. Instead, ICD-10-PCS provides a standardized level of specificity that can be predicted across the system.

Diagnosis Information Excluded – Another key feature of ICD-10-PCS is that information regarding a diagnosis is excluded from the code description. This is not true of ICD-9-CM which often contains diagnosis information in its procedures codes. Including diagnosis information within a procedure code limits the flexibility and functionality of a procedural coding system. It has the effect of placing a code "off limits" if the diagnosis in the medical record does not match the diagnosis in the procedure code description.

Diagnosis information is not contained in any ICD-10-PCS codes. The actual diagnoses codes, not the procedure codes, will specify the reason for the procedure.

NOS Code Options Restricted – ICD-9-CM often designates codes as "unspecified" or "not otherwise specified". In contrast, the standardized level of specificity of ICD-10-PCS restricts the use of broadly applicable NOS or unspecified code options. ICD-10-PCS requires a minimal level of specificity in order to construct a code.

Each character in ICD-10-PCS defines information about the procedure with all seven characters containing a specific value obtained from a single row of a table to build a valid code. Even values such as the sixth character value Z, no device, and the seventh character value Z, no qualifier, provide important information regarding the procedure performed.

Limited NEC Code Options – ICD-9-CM often designates codes as "not elsewhere classified" or "other specified" throughout the classification system. NEC options are provided in ICD-10-PCS, but only for specific, limited use.

In the Medical and Surgical section of ICD-10-PCS, two significant "not elsewhere classified" options are the root operation value Q, Repair and the device value Y, *other device.*

The root operation Repair is a true NEC value and is only used when the procedure performed is not one of the other 30 root operations in the Medical and Surgical section.

Other devices is intended to be used to temporarily define new devices that do not have a specific value assigned, until one can be added to the system. No categories of medical or surgical devices are permanently classified to *other devices.*

Source: CMS 2011b

Activity 2: Identifying Problems with ICD-9-CM Procedure Codes
Review and identify the problem with ICD-9-CM procedure codes for the following questions and then select the characteristic in ICD-10-PCS that address the problem.

1. 28.11, Biopsy of tonsils and adenoids
   a. NOS code option excluded
   b. Diagnosis information excluded
   c. Standardized terminology
   d. Standardized level of specificity

2. 51.22, Cholecystectomy
   a. NOS code option excluded
   b. Diagnosis information excluded
   c. Standardized terminology
   d. Standardized level of specificity

3. 38.91–38.99, Puncture of vessels, does not specify site whereas 38.00–38.09, Incision of vessel, provides fourth digit subclassification for specifying the vessel
   a. NOS code options excluded
   b. Diagnosis information excluded
   c. Standardized terminology
   d. Standardized level of specificity

4. 23.01, Extraction of deciduous tooth
   a. NOS code options excluded
   b. Diagnosis information excluded
   c. Standardized terminology
   d. Standardized level of specificity

5. 42.40, Esophagectomy, not otherwise specified
   a. NOS code options excluded
   b. Diagnosis information excluded
   c. Standardized terminology
   d. Standardized level of specificity

Activity 3: ICD-10-PCS Key Attribute – Completeness
Compare the following pairs of codes for drainage and identify the differences and similarities in the codes.

1. 0C9P00Z vs. 0B9100Z
2. 0B9300Z vs. 0B933ZX
3. 0H90X0Z vs. 0H90XZZ

Definitions Used in ICD-10-PCS

As previously mentioned, ICD-10-PCS has standardized, specific definitions and/or meanings for the “values” and characters.” Following are these definitions:

Character – One of the seven components that comprise an ICD-10-PCS procedure code

Value – Individual units defined for each character and represented by a number or letter

Procedure – The complete specification of the seven characters

Section (1st character) – Defines the general type of procedure

Body System (2nd character) – Defines the general physiological system on which the procedure is performed or anatomical region where the procedure is performed

Root Operation/Type (3rd character) – Defines the objective of the procedure

Body Part or Region (4th character) – Defines the specific anatomical site where the procedure is performed

Approach (5th character) – Defines the technique used to reach the site of the procedure

Device (6th character) – Defines the material or appliance that remains in or on the body at the end of the procedure

Qualifier (7th character) – Defines the additional attribute of the procedure performed, if applicable

Source: CMS 2011b

Having standard and strict definitions of terms in ICD-10-PCS provides clarity and makes the system easier to use. Let’s take an example of the term *resection* and see how having an exact definition to work from leads to consistent use and coding accuracy.

Sample definitions of the term *resection*:

Definition	**Source**
Cutting out or off, without replacement, all of the body part	ICD-10-PCS Reference Manual
The surgical removal of part of an organ or structure	*Merriam-Webster's Medical Dictionary*
1. A procedure performed for the specific purpose of removal, as in removal of articular ends of one or both bones forming a joint. 2. To remove a part. 3. Syn: excision	*Stedman's Medical Dictionary*
Removal of a portion or all of an organ or other structure. Called also excision and ectomy.	*Dorland's Illustrated Medical Dictionary*

As you can see, each of the medical dictionaries has a slightly different definition for resection. However, ICD-10-PCS has only one definition. Therefore, you would need to closely review the documentation in the medical record to ensure that the type of procedure being coded to the root operation "resection" meets the definition. If it does not, even though the physician may have called the procedure a resection, when classifying it in ICD-10-PCS it will be coded to a different root operation.

Example: Some examples of procedures classified to the root operation Resection are:

- Right hemicolectomy
- Total mastectomy
- Total lobectomy of lung
- Laparoscopic-assisted total vaginal hysterectomy

The resection definition is just one of many found in the Medical and Surgical section of ICD-10-PCS. It is important to become familiar with the definitions for all the root operations and approaches in order to correctly translate the procedures documented in the medical records into ICD-10-PCS codes.

To build upon the knowledge already gained regarding standardized terminology refer to Appendix B, "Root Operations," and Appendix C, "Approaches," located in this training manual and read through the definitions.

Note: Becoming familiar with these definitions is critical to success in ICD-10-PCS coding. Building codes correctly relies on the correct interpretation and understanding of these definitions.

Activity 4: Approach Definitions

For this activity you will select the correct approach value for each question.

1. Which approach value is defined as: "Entry, by puncture or minor incision, of instrumentation through the skin or mucous membrane and/or any other body layers necessary to reach the site of the procedure"?

2. Which approach value is defined as "Entry of instrumentation through a natural or artificial external opening to reach and visualize the site of the procedure, and entry, by puncture or minor incision, of instrumentation through the skin or mucous membrane and any other body layers necessary to aid in the performance of the procedure"?
3. Which approach value is defined as: "Entry, by puncture or minor incision of instrumentation through the skin or mucous membrane and/or any other body layers necessary to reach and visualize the site of the procedure"?
4. Which approach value is defined as: "Entry of instrumentation through a natural or artificial external opening to reach and visualize the site of the procedure"?

5. Which approach value is defined as: "Entry of instrumentation through a natural or artificial external opening to reach the site of the procedure"?

Section 2 Review Questions

1. Which of the following key attributes is the one that provides the framework for all other structural attributes?
    a. Multiaxial structure
    b. Completeness
    c. Expandability
    d. Standardized terminology

2. True or False? Every procedure that uses a different approach will have its own unique code.
    a. True
    b. False

3. Which of the following would you find in ICD-10-PCS?
    a. Combination codes
    b. Eponyms
    c. Information pertaining to a diagnosis in a code description
    d. Limited NEC code options

Section 3 – Review of Medical and Surgical Section – Section Value 0

Overview of the Medical and Surgical Section

In this section an overview of the Medical and Surgical section of ICD-10-PCS is provided. Additionally, this section briefly reviews the 31 ICD-10-PCS body system values and illustrates root operations that share similar attributes.

General Overview of the Medical and Surgical Section

The Medical and Surgical codes have a first character value of "0." Characters 2–7 represent body system, root operation, body part, approach, device, and qualifier. The following diagram summarizes the organizational structure of the Medical and Surgical section.

Character 1 Section	Character 2 Body System	Character 3 Root Operation	Character 4 Body Part	Character 5 Approach	Character 6 Device	Character 7 Qualifier

The Medical and Surgical section is by far the largest of the 16 sections of ICD-10-PCS.

Example: Some of the procedures found in this section are:

- Thrombectomy
- Lithotripsy
- Inguinal hernia repair
- Gastrostomy tube change
- Cardiac Mapping
- Insertion of central venous catheter

Body Systems

The meaning of the second character in the Medical and Surgical section is general body system. This character may be represented by one of thirty-one values, 0–9, B–D, F–H, J–N and P–Y. However, the way in which ICD-10-PCS defines a "body system" is a bit different than the usual meaning of the term. A review of the following list shows how some customary body systems are given multiple body-system values. For example, note the circulatory system does not have a single value.

Values	ICD-10-PCS Body Systems
0	Central Nervous System
1	Peripheral Nervous System
2	Heart and Great Vessels
3	Upper Arteries
4	Lower Arteries
5	Upper Veins
6	Lower Veins
7	Lymphatic and Hemic System
8	Eye
9	Ear, Nose, Sinus
B	Respiratory System
C	Mouth and Throat
D	Gastrointestinal System
F	Hepatobiliary System and Pancreas
G	Endocrine System
H	Skin and Breast
J	Subcutaneous Tissue and Fascia
K	Muscles
L	Tendons
M	Bursae and Ligaments
N	Head and Facial Bones
P	Upper Bones
Q	Lower Bones
R	Upper Joints
S	Lower Joints
T	Urinary System
U	Female Reproductive System
V	Male Reproductive System
W	Anatomic Region, General
X	Anatomical Region, Upper Extremities
Y	Anatomic Regions, Lower Extremities

Root Operations

The third character in the Medical and Surgical section is the root operation. There are a total of 31 root operations within this section and when coding you must select the root operation that matches the specific objective of the procedure as documented in the medical record. These 31 root operations are divided into nine groups that share similar attributes.

The nine groups are:

1. Procedures that take out some/all of a body part
2. Procedures that take out solids/fluids/gases from a body part
3. Procedures involving cutting or separation only
4. Procedures that put in/put back or move some/all of a body part
5. Procedures that alter the diameter/route of a tubular body part
6. Procedures that always involve a device
7. Procedures involving examination only
8. Procedures that define other repairs
9. Procedures that define objectives

The following table lists these nine groups and the root operations within each group.

Root Operation	What Operation Does	Objective of Procedure	Procedure Site	Example
Root operations that take out some/all of a body part				
Excision	Takes out some/all of a body part	Cutting out/off without replacement	Some of a body part	Breast lumpectomy
Resection	Takes out some/all of a body part	Cutting out/off without replacement	All of a body part	Total mastectomy
Detachment	Takes out some/all of a body part	Cutting out/off without replacement	Extremity only, any level	Amputation above elbow
Destruction	Takes out some/all of a body part	Eradicating without replacement	Some/all of a body part	Fulguration of endometrium
Extraction	Takes out some/all of a body part	Pulling out or off without replacement	Some/all of a body part	Suction D&C
Root operations that take out solids/fluids/gases from a body part				
Drainage	Takes out solids/fluids/gases from a body part	Taking/letting out fluids/gases	Within a body part	Incision and drainage
Extirpation	Takes out solids/fluids/gases from a body part	Taking/cuttin g out solid matter	Within a body part	Thrombectomy
Fragmentation	Takes out solids/fluids/gases from a body part	Breaking solid matter into pieces	Within a body part	Lithotripsy
Root operations involving cutting or separation only				
Division	Involves cutting or separation only	Cutting into/ separating a body part	Within a body part	Neurotomy
Release	Involves cutting or separation only	Freeing a body part from constraint	Around a body part	Adhesiolysis

Root operations that put in/put back or move some/all of a body part				
Transplantation	Puts in/puts back or moves some/all of a body part	Putting in a living body part from a person/ animal	Some/all of a body part	Kidney transplant
Reattachment	Puts in/puts back or moves some/all of a body part	Putting back a detached body part	Some/all of a body part	Reattach severed finger
Transfer	Puts in/puts back or moves some/all of a body part	Moving, to function for a similar body part	Some/all of a body part	Skin tissue transfer
Reposition	Puts in/puts back or moves some/all of a body part	Moving, to normal or other suitable location	Some/all of a body part	Move undescended testicle
Root operations that alter the diameter/route of a tubular body part				
Restriction	Alters the diameter/route of a tubular body part	Partially closing orifice/lumen	Tubular body part	Gastroesophageal fundoplication
Occlusion	Alters the diameter/route of a tubular body part	Completely closing orifice/lumen	Tubular body part	Fallopian tube ligation
Dilation	Alters the diameter/route of a tubular body part	Expanding orifice/ lumen	Tubular body part	Percutaneous transluminal coronary angioplasty (PTCA)
Bypass	Alters the diameter/route of a tubular body part	Altering route of passage	Tubular body part	Coronary artery bypass graft (CABG)
Root operations that always involve a device				
Insertion	Always involves a device	Putting in non-biological device	In/on a body part	Central line insertion
Replacement	Always involves a device	Putting in device that replaces a body part	Some/all of a body part	Total hip replacement
Supplement	Always involves a device	Putting in device that reinforces or augments a body part	In/on a body part	Abdominal wall herniorrhaphy using mesh
Change	Always involves a device	Exchanging a device without cutting/puncturing	In/on a body part	Drainage tube change

Removal	Always involves a device	Taking out device	In/on a body part	Central line removal
Revision	Always involves a device	Correcting a malfunctioning /displaced device	In/on a body part	Revision of pacemaker insertion
Root operations involving examination only				
Inspection	Involves examination only	Visual/manual exploration	Some/all of a body part	Diagnostic cystoscopy
Map	Involves examination only	Locating electrical impulses/ functional areas	Brain/ cardiac conduction mechanism	Cardiac eletrophysiological study
Root operations that include other repairs				
Repair	Includes other repairs	Restoring body part to its normal structure	Some/all of a body part	Suture laceration
Control	Includes other repair	Stopping/ attempting to stop post-procedural bleed	Anatomical region	Post-prostatectomy bleeding
Root operations that include other objectives				
Fusion	Includes other objectives	Rending joint immobile	Joint	Spinal fusion
Alteration	Includes other objectives	Modifying body part for cosmetic purposes without affecting function	Some/all of a body part	Face lift
Creation	Includes other objectives	Making new structure for sex change operation	Perineum	Artificial vagina/ penis

Activity 5: Root Operations

Complete the following sentences with the correct root operation

1. Cutting off all or a portion of an extremity is the definition of ____________.
2. Cutting out or off, without replacement, a portion of a body part is the definition of ____________.
3. Taking out or off a device from a body part is the definition of ____________.
4. Correcting, to the extent possible, a malfunctioning or displaced device is the definition of ____________.
5. Pulling or stripping out or off all or a portion of a body part by the use of force is the definition of ____________.

Code Components: Body Part, Approach, Device, and Qualifier

Body Part

The meaning of the fourth character in the Medical and Surgical section is body part. The value chosen for this character represents the specific part of the body system (character 2) on which the surgery was performed. Body parts may specify laterality. Some examples of body parts and their body systems in ICD-10-PCS are:

Body System	Body Part
Lower extremities	Left foot
Central nervous	Trigeminal nerve
Upper veins	Right cephalic vein
Gastrointestinal	Stomach

ICD-10-PCS does not provide a specific value for every body part. In those instances the body part value selected would be either the whole body part value (for example, alveolar process is part of the mandible), or in the instance of nerves and vessels, the body part value is coded to the closest proximal branch.

To further your understanding in the selection of the appropriate body part, review Appendix A, "Body Part Key by Anatomical Term," located in the back of the training manual.

Approach

ICD-10-PCS defines *approach* as the technique used to reach the site of the procedure. It is important to know the differences between the different approaches in order to correctly assign the fifth character value in the Medical and Surgical section.

There are seven different approaches, as shown in the table. The approach is comprised of three components: the access location, method and type of instrumentation.

Access Location – For procedures performed on an internal body part, the access location specifies the external site through which the site of the procedure is reached. There are two general types of access locations: skin or mucous membranes and external orifices. Every approach value, except external, includes one of these two access locations. The skin or mucous membrane can be cut or punctured to reach the procedure site and all open and percutaneous approach values use this access location. The site of a procedure can also be reached through an external opening which can be either natural (e.g., mouth) or artificial (e.g., colostomy stoma).

Method – For procedures performed on an internal body part, the method specifies how the external access location is entered. An open method specifies cutting through the skin or mucous membrane and any other intervening body layers necessary to expose the site of the procedure. An instrumentation method specifies the entry of instrumentation through the access location to the internal procedure site. Instrumentation can be introduced by puncture or minor incision, or through an external opening.

Type of Instrumentation – For procedures performed on an internal body part, instrumentation refers to the specialized equipment used to perform the procedure. Instrumentation is used in all internal approaches other than the basic open approach. Instrumentation may or may not include the capacity to visualize the procedure site. For example, the instrumentation used to perform a sigmoidoscopy permits the internal site of the procedure to be visualized, while the instrumentation used to perform a needle biopsy of the liver does not. The term "endoscopic" as used in approach values refers to instrumentation that permits a site to be visualized.

Procedures performed directly on the skin or mucous membrane are identified by the external approach. Procedures performed indirectly by the application of external force are also identified by the external approach (e.g., closed fracture reduction)

Approach	**Definition**
Open	Cutting through the skin or mucous membrane and any other body layers necessary to expose the site of the procedure
Percutaneous	Entry, by puncture or minor incision, of instrumentation through the skin or mucous membrane and/or any other body layers necessary to reach the site of the procedure
Percutaneous Endoscopic	Entry, by puncture or minor incision, of instrumentation through the skin or mucous membrane and/or any other body layers necessary to reach and visualize the site of the procedure
Via Natural or Artificial Opening	Entry of instrumentation through a natural or artificial external opening to reach the site of the procedure
Via Natural or Artificial Opening Endoscopic	Entry of instrumentation through a natural or artificial external opening to reach and visualize the site of the procedure

Via Natural or Artificial Opening Endoscopic with Percutaneous Endoscopic Assistance	Entry of instrumentation through a natural or artificial external opening to reach and visualize the site of the procedure, and entry, by puncture or minor incision, of instrumentation through the skin or mucous membrane and any other body layers necessary to aid in the performance of the procedure
External	Procedures performed directly on the skin or mucous membrane and procedures performed indirectly by the application of external force through the skin or mucous membrane

Source: CMS 2011a.

APPROACH VALUES

0 Open
3 Percutaneous
4 Percutaneous Endoscopic
7 Via Natural or Artificial Opening
8 Via Natural or Artificial Opening Endoscopic
F Via Natural or Artificial Opening with Percutaneous Endoscopic Assistance
X External

Activity 6: Medical and Surgical Approaches

1. The approach is comprised on three components: the access location, type of instrumentation, and ____________.
2. External approaches are performed directly on the mucous membrane or ____________.
3. What value is assigned for a percutaneous approach?
4. What approach value would be used when instruments are introduced through a natural opening to reach the site of the procedure?

Device and Qualifier

In the Medical and Surgical section the sixth character specifies devices that remain after the procedure is completed. The seventh character, qualifier, is used with certain procedures to define an additional attribute of the procedure. The following lists illustrate examples of the sixth and seventh characters available in the urinary system.

Device – Character 6

0 Drainage Device
2 Monitoring Device
3 Infusion Device
7 Autologous Tissue Substitute
C Extraluminal Device
D Intraluminal Device
J Synthetic Substitute
K Nonautologous Tissue Substitute
L Artificial Sphincter
M Stimulator Lead
Y Other Device
Z No Device

Qualifier – Character 7

0 Allogeneic
1 Syngeneic
2 Zooplastic
3 Kidney Pelvis, Right
4 Kidney Pelvis, Left
6 Ureter, Right
7 Ureter, Left
8 Colon
9 Colocutaneous
A Ileum
B Bladder
C Ileocutaneous
D Cutaneous
X Diagnostic
Z No Qualifier

Device – As previously mentioned, the device is specified in the sixth character and is only used to specify devices that remain after the procedure is completed. There are four general types of devices:

- Biological or synthetic material that takes the place of all or a portion of a body part (i.e., skin graft, joint prosthesis)
- Biological or synthetic material that assists or prevents a physiological function (i.e., IUD)
- Therapeutic material that is not absorbed by, eliminated by, or incorporated into a body part (i.e., radioactive implant)
- Mechanical or electronic appliances used to assist, monitor, take the place of or prevent a physiological function (i.e., cardiac defibrillator, orthopedic pin)

Instrumentation used to visualize the procedure site is not specified in the device value. This information is specified in the approach value.

If the objective of the procedure is to put in a device, then the root operation is Insertion. If the device is put in to meet an objective other than Insertion, the root operation defining the underlying objective of the procedure is used, with the device specified in the sixth character, device. For example, if a procedure to replace the hip joint is performed, the root operation Replacement is coded and the prosthetic device is specified as the sixth character. Materials incidental to a procedure such as clips, ligatures and sutures are not specified in the device character.

Qualifier – The seventh character specifies the qualifier which contains unique values for individual procedures as needed. For example, the qualifier can be used to identify the destination site in a bypass.

Source: CMS 2011a

Activity 7: Coding Exercise

Using the ICD-10-PCS Index and Tables, assign the correct code for the following:

1. Diagnostic EGD with gastric biopsy
2. Laparoscopic total cholecystectomy
3. Left partial mastectomy, open
4. Open left femoral-popliteal artery bypass using cadaver vein graft

Section 3 Review Questions

1. Which of the following body systems is assigned multiple body-system values in ICD-10-PCS?
   a. Urinary System
   b. Respiratory System
   c. Musculoskeletal System
   d. Gastrointestinal System

2. Which of the following root operations does not share similar attributes with the other three root operations and therefore is not within the same group?
   a. Removal
   b. Excision
   c. Resection
   d. Destruction

3. True or False? The meaning of the second character in the Medical and Surgical section is body part.
   a. True
   b. False

Section 4 – Review of the Medical and Surgical-related Sections – Section Values 1–9

Organization and Classification of Medical and Surgical-related Sections

General Overview of the Medical and Surgical-related Sections

The Medical and Surgical-related procedure codes have a first character value of 1–9. For the remaining character definitions, some of those from the Medical and Surgical section apply but variations do exist.

To become familiar with the general differences, compare the code structure of the Obstetrics section, which carries the same meaning for all seven characters as those in the Medical and Surgical section, with the other Medical and Surgical-related sections.

> **Note:** Keep in mind while the general description may be the same, the actual detail may not be.

> *Example:* Ten of the 12 root operations found in the Obstetrics section are also in the Medical and Surgical section. There are also two additional root operations unique to Obstetrics.

Obstetrics – Section Value 1

Character 1 Section	Character 2 Body System	Character 3 Root Operation	Character 4 Body Part	Character 5 Approach	Character 6 Device	Character 7 Qualifier

Placement – Section Value 2

Character 1 Section	Character 2 Body System	Character 3 Root Operation	Character 4 Body Region	Character 5 Approach	Character 6 Device	Character 7 Qualifier

Administration – Section Value 3

Character 1 Section	Character 2 Body System	Character 3 Root Operation	Character 4 Body System	Character 5 Approach	Character 6 Substance	Character 7 Qualifier

Measurement and Monitoring – Section Value 4

Character 1 Section	Character 2 Body System	Character 3 Root Operation	Character 4 Body System	Character 5 Approach	Character 6 Function	Character 7 Qualifier

Extracorporeal Assistance and Performance – Section Value 5

Character 1 Section	Character 2 Body System	Character 3 Root Operation	Character 4 Body System	Character 5 Duration	Character 6 Function	Character 7 Qualifier

Extracorporeal Therapies – Section Value 6

Character 1 Section	Character 2 Body System	Character 3 Root Operation	Character 4 Body System	Character 5 Duration	Character 6 Qualifier	Character 7 Qualifier

Osteopathic – Section Value 7

Character 1 Section	Character 2 Body System	Character 3 Root Operation	Character 4 Body Region	Character 5 Approach	Character 6 Method	Character 7 Qualifier

Other Procedures – Section Value 8

Character 1 Section	Character 2 Body System	Character 3 Root Operation	Character 4 Body Region	Character 5 Approach	Character 6 Method	Character 7 Qualifier

Chiropractic – Section Value 9

Character 1 Section	Character 2 Body System	Character 3 Root Operation	Character 4 Body Region	Character 5 Approach	Character 6 Method	Character 7 Qualifier

Examples of Procedures Found in the Medical and Surgical-related Sections

Now that you have an idea of the character values for the various Medical and Surgical-related sections, the next step is to understand the types of procedures found in each section. To assist you, two examples from each section are presented next.

Section	Examples
Obstetrics	Manually-assisted delivery Laparoscopy with total excision of tubal pregnancy
Placement	Application of sterile dressing to neck wound Change of vaginal packing
Administration	Epidural injection of mixed steroid and local anesthetic for pain control Peritoneal dialysis via indwelling catheter
Measurement and Monitoring	Holter monitoring Fetal heart rate monitoring, transvaginal
Extracorporeal Assistance and Performance	Controlled mechanical ventilation, 50 hours Cardiopulmonary bypass in conjunction with CABG
Extracorporeal Therapies	Plasmapheresis, single treatment Whole body hypothermia, single treatment
Osteopathic	Indirect osteopathic treatment of pelvis Isotonic muscle energy treatment of left arm
Other Procedures	Robotic assisted open prostatectomy CT computer assisted sinus surgery
Chiropractic	Chiropractic treatment of lumbar region using short lever specific contact Chiropractic extra-articular treatment of knees

Code Components and Coding Tips – Section Values 1–9

Obstetrics, Placement, and Administration Sections

Obstetrics Section – The Obstetrics section follows the same conventions established in the Medical and Surgical section, with all seven characters retaining the same meaning. Obstetrics procedure codes have a first character value of 1 and the second character value for body system is Pregnancy. There are a total of 12 root operations in the Obstetrics section. Ten of these, Change, Drainage, Extraction, Insertion, Inspection, Removal, Repair, Reposition, Resection and Transplantation are also found in the Medical and Surgical section. The Obstetrics section also includes two additional root operations unique to this section.

Value	Description	Definition
A	Abortion	Artificially terminating a pregnancy
E	Delivery	Assisting the passage of the products of conception from the genital canal

Abortion is subdivided according to whether an additional device such as laminaria or abortifacient is used, or whether the abortion was performed by mechanical means.

Delivery applies only to manually-assisted vaginal delivery and is defined as assisting the passage of the products of conception from the genital canal.
A cesarean section is not its own unique root operation, because the underlying objective is Extraction (pulling out all or a portion of a body part).

The body part values in the Obstetrics section are:

- Products of conception
- Products of conception, retained
- Products of conception, ectopic

Only procedures performed on the products of conception are included in the Obstetrics section; procedures performed on the pregnant female are coded in the Medical and Surgical section (i.e., episiotomy). The term “products of conception” refers to all physical components of a pregnancy, including the fetus, amnion, umbilical cord and placenta.

The fifth character specifies approaches and the sixth character is used for devices such as fetal monitoring electrodes. Qualifier values are specific to root operation, and are used to specify the type of extraction (i.e., low forceps, low cervical cesarean, etc), the type of fluid taken out during a drainage procedure (i.e., amniotic fluid, fetal blood, etc.) or the body system of the products of conception on which the repair was performed.

Placement Section – Placement section codes represent procedures for putting an externally placed device in or on a body region for the purpose of protection, immobilization, stretching, compression or packing. Codes from this section have a first character value of 2. The second character value for body system is either anatomical regions or anatomical orifices. The root operations in the Placement section include only those procedures performed without making an incision or puncture. The root operations Change and Removal are contained in the Placement section, and retain the same meaning as in the Medical and Surgical section. The Placement section also includes five additional root operations, defined as follows:

Value	Description	Definition
1	Compression	Putting pressure on a body part
2	Dressing	Putting material on a body region for protection
3	Immobilization	Limiting or preventing motion of a body region
4	Packing	Putting material in a body region
6	Traction	Exerting a pulling force on a body region in a distal direction

The fourth character values are either body regions (i.e., chest wall, face, left upper leg) or natural orifices (i.e., ear, mouth and pharynx, urethra). Since all placement procedures are performed directly on the skin or mucus membrane, or performed indirectly by the application of external force through the skin or mucous membrane, the approach value is always External, character value X.

The sixth character, the device character always (except in the case of manual traction) specifies the device placed during the procedure (i.e., cast, splint, bandage, etc.). Except for casts, devices in the placement section are off the shelf and do not require any extensive design, fabrication or fitting. The placement of devices that require extensive design, fabrication or fitting are coded in the Rehabilitation section of ICD-10-PCS. The qualifier character is not specified in this section; thus the qualifier value is always Z, no qualifier.

Administration Section – The Administration section includes infusions, injections and transfusions, as well as other related procedures, such as irrigation and tattooing. All codes in this section define procedures where a diagnostic or therapeutic substance is given to the patient.

Administrative procedures have a first character value of 3. The body system character for this section contains three values: circulatory system, indwelling device, and physiological systems and anatomical regions.

The three root operations in this section are classified according to the broad category of substance administered. If the substance given is a blood product or a cleansing substance, the procedure is coded to Transfusion and Irrigation, respectively. All other substances administered are coded to the root operation, Introduction. Following are the definitions for these three root operations:

Value	Description	Definition
0	Introduction	Putting in or on a therapeutic, diagnostic, nutritional, physiological, or prophylactic substance except blood or blood products
1	Irrigation	Putting in or on a cleansing substance
2	Transfusion	Putting in blood or blood products

The fourth character specifies the body system or region which identifies the site where the substance is administered, not the site where the substance administered takes effect. Sites include skin and mucous membrane, subcutaneous tissue and muscle which differentiate intradermal, subcutaneous and intramuscular injections respectively. Other sites include eye, respiratory tract, peritoneal cavity and epidural space.

The fifth character specifies approach with the approach for intradermal, subcutaneous and intramuscular introductions (i.e., injections) being percutaneous. If a catheter is placed to introduce a substance into an internal site within the circulatory system, then the approach is also percutaneous.
The body systems/regions for arteries and veins are peripheral artery, central artery, peripheral vein and central vein. The peripheral artery or vein is typically used when a substance is introduced locally into an artery or vein and in general, the substance introduced has a system effect.

The central artery or vein is typically used when the site where the substance is introduced is distant from the point of entry into the artery or vein and in general the substance introduced into a central artery or vein has a local effect.

The sixth character specifies the substance being introduced. Broad categories are defined, such as anesthetic, contrast, dialysate and blood products such as platelets. The seventh character, the qualifier, is used to indicate whether a substance transfused is autologous or nonautologous, or to further specify a substance introduced.

Source: CMS 2011a; CMS 2011b

Measurement and Monitoring, Extracorporeal Assistance and Performance, and Extracorporeal Therapies Sections

The Measurement and Monitoring, Extracorporeal Assistance and Performance, and Extracorporeal Therapies sections have similar general second through seventh character components, as shown here.

Measurement and Monitoring – Section Value 4

Character 1 Section	Character 2 Body System	Character 3 Root Operation	Character 4 Body System	Character 5 Approach	Character 6 Function	Character 7 Qualifier

Extracorporeal Assistance and Performance – Section Value 5

Character 1 Section	Character 2 Body System	Character 3 Root Operation	Character 4 Body System	Character 5 Duration	Character 6 Function	Character 7 Qualifier

Extracorporeal Therapies – Section Value 6

Character 1 Section	Character 2 Body System	Character 3 Root Operation	Character 4 Body System	Character 5 Duration	Character 6 Qualifier	Character 7 Qualifier

However, what the individual characters specify is dependent on the section from which you are coding.

Example: The body system is shown as the meaning for character 4.

Looking further into the specific definitions for this term in each section reveals the following:

Section	What the Fourth Character Specifies
Measurement and Monitoring	Body system measured or monitored
Extracorporeal Assistance and Performance	Body system to which extracorporeal assistance or performance is applied
Extracorporeal Therapies	Body system on which the extracorporeal therapy is performed

---

Measurement and Monitoring Section – Measurement and Monitoring section codes represent procedures for determining the level of a physiological or physical function. Procedure codes from this section have a first character value of 4 and the second character value for body system is either physiological systems (A) or physiological devices (B). There are two root operations in this section, as defined here:

Value	Description	Definition
0	Measurement	Determining the level of a physiological or physical function at a point in time
1	Monitoring	Determining the level of physiological or physical function repetitively over a period of time

The fourth character defines the body system measured or monitored. The fifth character specifies approaches as defined in the Medical and Surgical section. The sixth character specifies the physiological or physical function being measured or monitored. Examples of sixth character values in this section are conductivity, metabolism, pulse, temperature and volume. If a device used to perform the measurement or monitoring is inserted and left in, insertion of the device is coded as a separate procedure. The seventh character, qualifier, contains specific values as needed to further specify the body part or a variation of the procedure performed.

Extracorporeal Assistance and Performance Section – This section includes procedures performed in a critical care setting, such as mechanical ventilation and cardioversion. Additionally, this section includes procedures such as hemodialysis and hyperbaric oxygen therapy. Procedures from this section use equipment to support a physiological function in some way, whether it is breathing, circulating the blood or restoring the natural rhythm of the heart.

Extracorporeal Assistance and Performance codes have a first character value of 5. The second character of codes from this section is physiological systems.

There are three root operations in the Extracorporeal Assistance and Performance section, as specified here:

Value	Description	Definition
0	Assistance	Taking over a portion of a physiological function by extracorporeal means
1	Performance	Completely taking over a physiological function by extracorporeal means
2	Restoration	Returning, or attempting to return, a physiological function to its original state by extracorporeal means

The root operation Restoration contains a single procedure code that identifies extracorporeal cardioversion. The fourth character specifies the body system to which extracorporeal assistance or performance is applied and the fifth character specifies the duration of the procedure. For respiratory ventilation assistance or performance, the duration is specified in hours, i.e., <24 hours, 24-96 hours or >96 hours. The sixth character defines the physiological function assisted or performed (i.e., ventilation, oxygenation) and the seventh character defines the equipment used, if applicable.

Extracorporeal Therapies Section – The Extracorporeal Therapies section describes other extracorporeal procedures that are not defined by Assistance and Performance in section 5. Examples are bili-lite phototherapy and apheresis.

Codes from this section have a first character value of 6 and the second character value contains a single general body system, physiological systems. There are 10 root operations in this section, as defined below:

Value	Description	Definition
0	Atmospheric Control	Extracorporeal control of atmospheric pressure and composition
1	Decompression	Extracorporeal elimination of undissolved gas from body fluids
2	Electromagnetic Therapy	Extracorporeal treatment by electromagnetic rays
3	Hyperthermia	Extracorporeal raising of body temperature
4	Hypothermia	Extracorporeal lowering of body temperature
5	Pheresis	Extracorporeal separation of blood products
6	Phototherapy	Extracorporeal treatment by light rays
7	Ultrasound Therapy	Extracorporeal treatment by ultrasound
8	Ultraviolet Light Therapy	Extracorporeal treatment by ultraviolet light
9	Shock Wave Therapy	Extracorporeal treatment by shock waves

The fourth character of codes from this section specifies the body system on which the extracorporeal therapy is performed (i.e., skin, circulatory) and the fifth character defines the duration of the procedure (i.e., single, intermittent). The sixth character is not specified for extracorporeal therapies and always has a character value of Z, no qualifier. The seventh character is used in the root operation Pheresis to specify the blood component on which the pheresis is performed.

Source: CMS 2011a; CMS 2011b

Osteopathic, Other Procedures, and Chiropractic Sections

As illustrated below, the Osteopathic, Other Procedures, and Chiropractic sections also are very analogous at the general description level of the second through seventh character components.

Osteopathic – Section Value 7

Character 1 Section	Character 2 Body System	Character 3 Root Operation	Character 4 Body Region	Character 5 Approach	Character 6 Method	Character 7 Qualifier

Other Procedures – Section Value 8

Character 1 Section	Character 2 Body System	Character 3 Root Operation	Character 4 Body Region	Character 5 Approach	Character 6 Method	Character 7 Qualifier

Chiropractic – Section Value 9

Character 1 Section	Character 2 Body System	Character 3 Root Operation	Character 4 Body Region	Character 5 Approach	Character 6 Method	Character 7 Qualifier

---

Osteopathic Section – Section 7, Osteopathic, is one of the smallest sections in ICD-10-PCS. Procedures codes from this section have a first character value of 7 and a single body system, anatomical regions (W). Additionally, there is only one root operation in the Osteopathic section, Treatment.

Value	Description	Definition
0	Treatment	Manual treatment to eliminate or alleviate somatic dysfunction and related disorders

The fourth character defines the body region on which the osteopathic manipulation is performed. The fifth character value, approach, is always External in this section. The sixth character specifies the method by which the manipulation is accomplished. The seventh character is not specified in the Osteopathic section and always has the value, No Qualifier (Z).

Other Procedures Section – The Other Procedures section contains codes for procedures not included in the other Medical and Surgical-related sections such as suture removal, acupuncture and in vitro fertilization. Codes in this section have a first character value of 8. There is a single body system for this section, physiological systems and anatomical regions (E). A single root operation, Other Procedures, is found in this section, as defined here:

Value	Description	Definition
0	Other Procedures	Methodologies which attempt to remediate or cure a disorder or disease

The fourth character identifies specific body region values. The fifth character defines the approach used to perform the procedure. The sixth character specifies the method (i.e., robotic assisted procedure) and the seventh character, qualifier, contains specific values as applicable.

Chiropractic Section – Chiropractic section procedure codes have a first character of 9. This section consists of a single body system, Anatomical Regions (W) for the second character value. Additionally, there is only one root operation in the Chiropractic section, as identified here:

Value	Description	Definition
B	Manipulation	Manual procedure that involves a directed thrust to move a joint past the physiological range of motion, without exceeding the anatomical limit

The fourth character specifies the body region on which the chiropractic manipulation is performed and the fifth character, approach, is always External (X). The sixth character is the method by which the manipulation is accomplished. The seventh character, qualifier, is not specified in the Chiropractic section, and always has the value No Qualifier (Z).

Source: CMS 2011a; CMS 2011b

Activity 8: Coding Exercise

Using the ICD-10-PCS Index and tables, assign the correct code for the following:

1. Percutaneous irrigation of knee joint
2. Laparoscopy with total excision of tubal pregnancy
3. Peritoneal dialysis via indwelling catheter
4. Intermittent mechanical ventilation, 24 consecutive hours

Activity 9: Root Operations in the Medical and Surgical-related Sections

1. Complete the following sentence. Putting material on a body region for protection is the definition of ___________.

2. Complete the following sentence. Determining the level of a physiological or physical function at a point in time is the definition of ___________.

3. Complete the following sentence. Completely taking over a physiological function by extracorporeal means is the definition of ___________.

4. Complete the following sentence. Extracorporeal lowering of body temperature is the definition of ___________.

5. Complete the following sentence. Putting in or on a cleansing substance is the definition of ___________.

Section 4 Review Questions

1. Which of the following procedures is assigned to the Medical and Surgical-related sections of ICD-10-PCS?
    a. Central line insertion
    b. Holter monitoring
    c. Central line removal
    d. Revision of pacemaker insertion

2. Which of the following code components is found only in the Medical and Surgical-related sections?
    a. Function
    b. Body System
    c. Qualifier
    d. Root Operation

3. True or False? Delivery is a root operation found in the Obstetrics section.
    a. True
    b. False

Section 5 – Review of Ancillary Sections – Section Values B–D and F–H

Organization and Classification of Ancillary Sections

General Overview of the Ancillary Sections

The Ancillary procedure codes have a first character value of B–D or F–H. For the remaining character definitions, only a few of those from the Medical and Surgical section apply. There are six Ancillary sections of ICD-10-PCS, as illustrated in the following table:

Section Value	Description
B	Imaging
C	Nuclear Medicine
D	Radiation Oncology
F	Physical Rehabilitation and Diagnostic Audiology
G	Mental Health
H	Substance Abuse Treatment

To become familiar with the general differences, compare the code structure of the Medical and Surgical section with the Ancillary sections. Keep in mind, while the general description may be the same, the actual detail may not be. For example, the Imaging section includes the characters body system and body part as does the Medical and Surgical section. However, the Imaging section defines value 3 as circulatory system, upper arteries (above diaphragm), but the circulatory system in the Medical and Surgical section is assigned multiple body system values.

Medical and Surgical – Section Value 0

Character 1 Section	Character 2 Body System	Character 3 Root Operation	Character 4 Body Part	Character 5 Approach	Character 6 Device	Character 7 Qualifier

Imaging – Section Value B

Character 1 Section	Character 2 Body System	Character 3 Root Type	Character 4 Body Part	Character 5 Contrast	Character 6 Qualifier	Character 7 Qualifier

Nuclear Medicine – Section Value C

Character 1 Section	Character 2 Body System	Character 3 Root Type	Character 4 Body Part	Character 5 Radionuclide	Character 6 Qualifier	Character 7 Qualifier

Radiation Oncology – Section Value D

Character 1 Section	Character 2 Body System	Character 3 Root Type	Character 4 Body Part	Character 5 Modality Qualifier	Character 6 Isotope	Character 7 Qualifier

Physical Rehabilitation and Diagnostic Audiology – Section Value F

Character 1 Section	Character 2 Section Qualifier	Character 3 Root Type	Character 4 Body System/ Region	Character 5 Type Qualifier	Character 6 Equipment	Character 7 Qualifier

Mental Health – Section Value G

Character 1 Section	Character 2 Body System	Character 3 Root Type	Character 4 Type Qualifier	Character 5 Qualifier	Character 6 Qualifier	Character 7 Qualifier

Substance Abuse Treatment – Section Value H

Character 1 Section	Character 2 Body System	Character 3 Root Type	Character 4 Type Qualifier	Character 5 Qualifier	Character 6 Qualifier	Character 7 Qualifier

Examples of Procedures Found in the Ancillary Sections

Now that you have an idea of the character values for the various Ancillary sections, the next step is to understand the types of procedures found in each section. To assist you, the following list presents two examples from each section.

Section	Examples
Imaging	Chest x-ray, AP/PA and lateral views Transrectal ultrasound of prostate gland
Nuclear Medicine	PET scan of myocardium using rubidium with dobutamine Gallium citrate scan of head and neck, single plane image
Radiation Oncology	Electron radiation treatment of right breast, dynamic 3-D with custom device Heavy particle radiation treatment of pancreas, 3 ports, custom device, four risk sites
Physical Rehabilitation and Diagnostic Audiology	Wound care treatment of left calf ulcer using pulsatile lavage Individual fitting of moveable brace, left knee
Mental Health	Crisis intervention, patient with severe mental disability Family psychotherapy with patient present
Substance Abuse Treatment	Substance abuse treatment planning Pharmacology treatment with Antabuse for drug addiction

Code Components and Coding Tips – Section Values B–D and F–H

Imaging, Nuclear Medicine, and Radiation Oncology Sections

Imaging Section – Imaging procedure codes have a first character value of B. Codes from this section represent procedures including plain radiography, fluoroscopy, CT, MRI and ultrasound. The second character of codes in this section defines the body system and the fourth character defines the specific body part. The third character identifies the root type of the imaging procedure, as defined in the following table.

Value	Description	Definition
0	Plain Radiography	Planar display of an image developed from the capture of external ionizing radiation on photographic or photoconductive plate
1	Fluoroscopy	Single plane or bi-plane real time display of an image developed from the capture of external ionizing radiation on a fluorescent screen. The image may also be stored by either digital or analog means.
2	Computerized Tomography (CT)	Computer reformatted digital display of multiplanar images developed from the capture of multiple exposures of external ionizing radiation
3	Magnetic Resonance Imaging (MRI)	Computer reformatted digital display of multiplanar images developed from the capture of radio-frequency signals emitted by nuclei in a body site excited within a magnetic field
4	Ultrasonography	Real time display of images of anatomy or flow information developed from the capture of reflected and attenuated high frequency sound waves

The fifth character specifies whether the contrast material used in the imaging procedure is high or low osmolar, when applicable. The sixth character qualifier provides further detail as needed, such as unenhanced followed by enhanced (image taken without contrast followed by an image with contrast). The seventh character is not specified in this section, and always has the value Z, none.

Nuclear Medicine – The Nuclear Medicine section is organized similar to the Imaging section. The only significant difference is in the character meaning of the fifth character. The codes in this section represent procedures that introduce radioactive material into the body in order to create an image, to diagnosis and treat pathologic conditions, or to assess metabolic functions.

Nuclear medicine procedure codes have a first character value of C and the second character specifies the body system on which the nuclear medicine procedure is performed. The third character, root type, indicates the type of nuclear medicine procedure, as defined in the following table:

Value	Description	Definition
1	Planar Nuclear Medicine Imaging	Introduction of radioactive materials into the body for single plane display of images developed from the capture of radioactive emissions
2	Tomographic (Tomo) Nuclear Medicine Imaging	Introduction of radioactive materials into the body for three-dimensional display of images developed from the capture of radioactive emissions
3	Positron Emission Tomography (PET)	Introduction of radioactive materials into the body for three-dimensional display of images developed from the simultaneous capture, 180 degrees apart, of radioactive emissions
4	Nonimaging Nuclear Medicine Uptake	Introduction of radioactive materials into the body for measurements of organ function, from the detection of radioactive emissions
5	Nonimaging Nuclear Medicine Probe	Introduction of radioactive materials into the body for the study of distribution and fate of certain substances by the detection of radioactive emissions from an external source
6	Nonimaging Nuclear Medicine Assay	Introduction of radioactive materials into the body for the study of body fluids and blood elements, by the detection of radioactive emissions
7	Systemic Nuclear Medicine Therapy	Introduction of unsealed radioactive materials into the body for treatment

The fourth character indicates the body part or body region studied with regional (i.e., lower extremity veins) and combination (i.e., liver and spleen) body part values being used. The fifth character defines the radionuclide, the radiation source. The sixth and seventh characters are not specified in this section, and always have the value Z, none.

Radiation Oncology Section – The Radiation Oncology section contains the radiation procedures performed for cancer treatment with the first character value of D. The second character of a code from this section specifies the body system. The third character defines the treatment modality as the root type. Four different root types are used in this section, as listed in this table.

Value	Description
0	Beam Radiation
1	Brachytherapy
2	Stereotactic Radiosurgery
Y	Other Radiation

The fourth character specifies the body part that is the focus of the radiation therapy. The fifth character further specifies treatment modality and the sixth character defines the radioactive isotope introduced into the body, if applicable. The seventh character is not specified in the Radiation Oncology section, and always has the value Z, none.

Source: CMS 2011a and CMS 2011b

Physical Rehabilitation and Diagnostic Audiology, Mental Health, and Substance Abuse Treatment Sections

The Physical Rehabilitation and Diagnostic Audiology, Mental Health, and Substance Abuse Treatment sections have some similar general second through seventh character components, as shown.

Physical Rehabilitation and Diagnostic Audiology – Section Value F

Character 1 Section	Character 2 Section Qualifier	Character 3 Root Type	Character 4 Body System/ Region	Character 5 Type Qualifier	Character 6 Equipment	Character 7 Qualifier

Mental Health – Section Value G

Character 1 Section	Character 2 Body System	Character 3 Root Type	Character 4 Type Qualifier	Character 5 Qualifier	Character 6 Qualifier	Character 7 Qualifier

Substance Abuse Treatment – Section Value H

Character 1 Section	Character 2 Body System	Character 3 Root Type	Character 4 Type Qualifier	Character 5 Qualifier	Character 6 Qualifier	Character 7 Qualifier

Example: The procedure type is shown as the meaning for character three for each of these three Ancillary sections.

Looking further into the specific definitions for this term (root type) in each of these three sections reveals the following:

Section	What the Character Named "Root Type" Specifies
Physical Rehabilitation and Diagnostic Audiology	One of 14 types – treatment, assessment fitting(s), or caregiver training
Mental Health	One of 11 types – namely, crisis intervention, family psychotherapy, biofeedback
Substance Abuse Treatment	One of 7 types – namely, detoxification, counseling, pharmacotherapy

Physical Rehabilitation and Diagnostic Audiology Section – Physical Rehabilitation section codes represent procedures including physical therapy, occupational therapy and speech-language pathology. Codes from this section have a first character value of F. The section qualifier rehabilitation or diagnostic audiology is specified in the second character. The third character specifies the 14 different root type values, as defined in the table.

Value	Description	Definition
0	Speech Assessment	Measurement of speech and related functions
1	Motor and/or Nerve Function Assessment	Measurement of motor, nerve and related functions
2	Activities of Daily Living Assessment	Measurement of functional level for activities of daily living
3	Hearing Assessment	Measurement of hearing and related functions
4	Hearing Aid Assessment	Measurement of the appropriateness and/or effectiveness of a hearing device
5	Vestibular Assessment	Measurement of the vestibular system and related functions
6	Speech Treatment	Application of techniques to improve, augment, or compensate for speech and related functional impairment
7	Motor Treatment	Exercise or activities to increase or facilitate motor function
8	Activities of Daily Living Treatment	Exercise or activities to facilitate functional competence for activities of daily living
9	Hearing Treatment	Application of techniques to improve, augment or compensate for hearing and related functional impairment
B	Hearing Aid Treatment	Application of techniques to improve the communication abilities of individuals with cochlear implant

C	Vestibular Treatment	Application of techniques to improve, augment, or compensate for vestibular and related functional impairment
D	Device Fitting	Fitting of a device designed to facilitate or support achievement of a higher level of function
F	Caregiver Training	Training in activities to support patient's optimal level of function

The root type Treatment includes training as well as activities which restore function. Treatment procedures include swallowing dysfunction exercises, bathing and showering techniques, wound management, gait training and a host of activities typically associated with rehabilitation. Assessments are further classified into more than one hundred different tests or methods. The majority of these assessments focus on the faculties of hearing and speech, but others focus on various aspects of body function and on the patient's quality of life.

The fourth character of codes from this section specifies the body region and/or system on which the procedure is performed. The fifth character is a type qualifier that further specifies the procedure performed and the sixth character specifies the equipment used. Specific equipment is not defined in the equipment value instead broad categories of equipment are specified. The seventh character is not specified in this section and always has the value Z, none.

Mental Health Section – Mental Health procedure codes have a first character value of G. The second character, body system, does not apply in this section and always has the value Z, none. The third character specifies the 11 root types, as listed in the table.

Value	Description
1	Psychological Tests
2	Crisis Intervention
5	Individual Psychotherapy
6	Counseling
7	Family Psychotherapy
B	Electroconvulsive Therapy
C	Biofeedback
F	Hypnosis
G	Narcosynthesis
H	Group Therapy
J	Light Therapy

The fourth character for codes in this section is a type qualifier. The fifth, sixth and seventh characters are not specified and always have the value Z, none.

Substance Abuse Treatment Section – Substance Abuse Treatment codes have a first character value of H. The second character, body system, does not apply in this section and always has the value Z, none. The third character specifies the seven root types, as defined in the table.

Value	Description
2	Detoxification Services
3	Individual Counseling
4	Group Counseling
5	Individual Psychotherapy
6	Family Counseling
8	Medication Management
9	Pharmacotherapy

The fourth character for codes in this section is a type qualifier. The fifth, sixth and seventh characters are not specified and always have the value Z, none.

Source: CMS 2011a and CMS 2011b

Section 5 Review Questions

1. Which of the following procedures is assigned to the Ancillary sections of ICD-10-PCS?
   a. Visual mobility test, single measurement
   b. Intermittent mechanical ventilation
   c. Routine fetal ultrasound, second trimester, twin gestation
   d. Peritoneal dialysis via indwelling catheter

2. Which of the following code components is found only in the Ancillary sections?
   a. Body system
   b. Qualifier
   c. Body part
   d. Isotope

3. True or False? Procedure codes found in the Ancillary sections have a first character value of B-D or F-H.
   a. True
   b. False

Section 6 – ICD-10-PCS Guidelines

With the development of a new classification comes the need to review content and decide what additional coding guidelines outside those available in the classification itself are necessary. The CMS has published draft general coding guidelines for coding professionals to follow in order to properly select an ICD-10-PCS code.

There are three main sections of guidelines:

A. Conventions
B. Medical and Surgical Section Guidelines (Section 0)
C. Obstetrics Section Guidelines (Section 1)

A. Conventions

A1. ICD-10-PCS codes are composed of seven characters. Each character is an axis of classification that specifies information about the procedure performed. Within a defined code range, a character specifies the same type of information in that axis of classification.

Example: The fifth axis of classification specifies the approach in sections 0 through 4 and 7 through 9 of the system.

A2. One of 34 possible values can be assigned to each axis of classification in the seven-character code: they are the numbers 0 through 9 and the alphabet (except I and O because they are easily confused with the numbers 1 and 0). The number of unique values used in an axis of classification differs as needed.

Example: Where the fifth axis of classification specifies the approach, seven different approach values are currently used to specify the approach.

A3. The valid values for an axis of classification can be added to as needed.

Example: If a significantly distinct type of device is used in a new procedure, a new device value can be added to the system.

A4. As with words in their context, the meaning of any single value is a combination of its axis of classification and any preceding values on which it may be dependent.

Example: The meaning of a body part value in the Medical and Surgical section is always dependent on the body system value. The body part value 0 in the Central Nervous body system specifies Brain and the body part value 0 in the Peripheral Nervous body system specifies Cervical Plexus.

A5. As the system is expanded to become increasingly detailed, over time more values will depend on preceding values for their meaning.

Example: In the Lower Joints body system, the device value 3 in the root operation Insertion specifies Infusion Device and the device value 3 in the root operation Fusion specifies Interbody Fusion Device.

A6. The purpose of the alphabetic index is to locate the appropriate table that contains all information necessary to construct a procedure code. The PCS Tables should always be consulted to find the most appropriate valid code.

A7. It is not required to consult the index first before proceeding to the Tables to complete the code. A valid code may be chosen directly from the Tables.

A8. All seven characters must be specified to be a valid code. If the documentation is incomplete for coding purposes, the physician should be queried for the necessary information.

A9. Within a PCS Table, valid codes include all combinations of choices in characters 4 through 7 contained in the same row of the table. In the following example, 0JHT3VZ is a valid code, and 0JHW3VZ is *not* a valid code.

Section: **0: Medical and Surgical**
Body System: **J: Subcutaneous Tissue and Fascia**
Operation: **H: Insertion:** Putting in a nonbiological appliance that monitors, assists, performs, or prevents a physiological function but does not physically take the place of a body part

Body Part	Approach	Device	Qualifier
S Subcutaneous Tissue and Fascia, Head and Neck **V** Subcutaneous Tissue and Fascia, Upper Extremity **W** Subcutaneous Tissue and Fascia, Lower Extremity	**0** Open **3** Percutaneous	**1** Radioactive Element **3** Infusion Device	**Z** No Qualifier
T Subcutaneous Tissue and Fascia, Trunk	**0** Open **3** Percutaneous	**1** Radioactive Element **3** Infusion Device **V** Infusion Pump	**Z** No Qualifier

A10. “And,” when used in a code description, means “and/or.”

Example: Lower Arm and Wrist Muscle means lower arm and/or wrist muscle.

A11. Many of the terms used to construct PCS codes are defined within the system. It is the coder's responsibility to determine what the documentation in the medical record equates to in the PCS definitions. The physician is not expected to use the terms used in PCS code descriptions, nor is the coder required to query the physician when the correlation between the documentation and the defined PCS terms is clear.

Example: When the physician documents "partial resection" the coder can independently correlate "partial resection" to the root operation Excision without querying the physician for clarification.

Source: CMS 2011b

Section-Specific Coding Guidelines

In addition to the coding conventions, CMS has developed two section specific guidelines; Medical and Surgical section guidelines and Obstetrics section guidelines.

Medical and Surgical Section (Section 0) Guidelines

B2. Body System Guidelines

General Guidelines

B2.1a. The procedure codes in the general anatomical regions body systems should only be used when the procedure is performed on an anatomical region rather than a specific body part (for example, root operations Control and Detachment, drainage of a body cavity) or on the rare occasion when no information is available to support assignment of a code to a specific body part.

Example: Control of postoperative hemorrhage is coded to the root operation Control found in the general anatomical regions body systems.

B2.1b. Body systems designated as upper or lower contain body parts located above or below the diaphragm respectively.

Example: Vein body parts above the diaphragm are found in the Upper Veins body system; vein body parts below the diaphragm are found in the Lower Veins body system.

B3. Root Operation Guidelines

General Guidelines

B3.1a. In order to determine the appropriate root operation, the full definition of the root operation as contained in the PCS Tables must be applied.

B3.1b. Components of a procedure specified in the root operation definition and explanation are not coded separately. Procedural steps necessary to reach the operative site and close the operative site are also not coded separately.

Example: Resection of a joint as part of a joint replacement procedure is included in the root operation definition of Replacement and is not coded separately. Laparotomy performed to reach the site of an open liver biopsy is not coded separately.

Multiple Procedures

B3.2. During the same operative episode, multiple procedures are coded if:

a. The same root operation is performed on different body parts as defined by distinct values of the body part character.

   Example: Diagnostic excision of liver and pancreas are coded separately.

b. The same root operation is repeated at different body sites that are included in the same body part value.

   Example: Excision of the sartorius muscle and excision of the gracilis muscle are both included in the upper leg muscle body part value, and multiple procedures are coded.

c. Multiple root operations with distinct objectives are performed on the same body part.

   Example: Destruction of sigmoid lesion and bypass of sigmoid colon are coded separately.

d. The intended root operation is attempted using one approach, but is converted to a different approach.

   Example: Laparoscopic cholecystectomy converted to an open cholecystectomy is coded as percutaneous endoscopic Inspection and open Resection.

Discontinued Procedures

B3.3. If the intended procedure is discontinued, code the procedure to the root operation performed. If a procedure is discontinued before any other root operation is performed, code the root operation Inspection of the body part or anatomical region inspected.

Example: A planned aortic valve replacement procedure is discontinued after the initial thoracotomy and before any incision is made in the heart muscle, when the patient becomes hemodynamically unstable. This procedure is coded as an open Inspection of the mediastinum.

Biopsy Followed by more Definitive Treatment

B3.4. If a diagnostic Excision, Extraction, or Drainage procedure (biopsy) is followed by a more definitive procedure, such as Destruction, Excision or Resection at the same procedure site, both the biopsy and the more definitive treatment are coded.

Example: Biopsy of breast followed by partial mastectomy at the same procedure site, both the biopsy and the partial mastectomy procedure are coded.

Overlapping Body Layers

B3.5. If the root operations Excision, Repair or Inspection are performed on overlapping layers of the musculoskeletal system, the body part specifying the deepest layer is coded.

Example: Excisional debridement that includes skin and subcutaneous tissue and muscle is coded to the muscle body part.

Bypass Procedures

B3.6a. Bypass procedures are coded by identifying the body part bypassed "from" and the body part bypassed "to." The fourth character body part specifies the body part bypassed from, and the qualifier specifies the body part bypassed to.

Example: Bypass from stomach to jejunum, stomach is the body part and jejunum is the qualifier.

B3.6b. Coronary arteries are classified by number of distinct sites treated, rather than number of coronary arteries or anatomic name of a coronary artery (for example, left anterior descending). Coronary artery bypass procedures are coded differently than other bypass procedures as described in the previous guideline. Rather than identifying the body part bypassed from, the body part identifies the number of coronary artery sites bypassed to, and the qualifier specifies the vessel bypassed from.

Example: Aortocoronary artery bypass of one site on the left anterior descending coronary artery and one site on the obtuse marginal coronary artery is classified in the body part axis of classification as two coronary artery sites and the qualifier specifies the aorta as the body part bypassed from.

B3.6c. If multiple coronary artery sites are bypassed, a separate procedure is coded for each coronary artery site that uses a different device and/or qualifier.

Example: Aortocoronary artery bypass and internal mammary coronary artery bypass are coded separately.

Control vs. More Definitive Root Operations

B3.7. The root operation Control is defined as, "Stopping, or attempting to stop, postprocedural bleeding." If an attempt to stop postprocedural bleeding is initially unsuccessful, and to stop the bleeding requires performing any of the definitive root operations Bypass, Detachment, Excision, Extraction, Reposition, Replacement, or Resection, then that root operation is coded instead of Control.

Example: Resection of spleen to stop postprocedural bleeding is coded to Resection instead of Control.

Excision vs. Resection

B3.8. PCS contains specific body parts for anatomical subdivisions of a body part, such as lobes of the lungs or liver and regions of the intestine. Resection of the specific body part is coded whenever all of the body part is cut out or off, rather than coding Excision of a less specific body part.

Example: Left upper lung lobectomy is coded to Resection of Upper Lung Lobe, Left rather than Excision of Lung, Left.

B3.9. If an autograft is obtained from a different body part in order to complete the objective of the procedure, a separate procedure is coded.

Example: Coronary bypass with excision of saphenous vein graft, excision of saphenous vein is coded separately.

Fusion Procedures of the Spine

B3.10a. The body part coded for a spinal vertebral joint(s) rendered immobile by a spinal fusion procedure is classified by the level of the spine (for example, thoracic). There are distinct body part values for a single vertebral joint and for multiple vertebral joints at each spinal level.

Example: Body part values specify Lumbar Vertebral Joint, Lumbar Vertebral Joints, 2 or More and Lumbosacral Vertebral Joint.

B3.10b. If multiple vertebral joints are fused, a separate procedure is coded for each vertebral joint that uses a different device and/or qualifier.

Example: Fusion of lumbar vertebral joint, posterior approach, anterior column and fusion of lumbar vertebral joint, posterior approach, posterior column are coded separately.

B3.10c. Combinations of devices and materials are often used on a vertebral joint to render the joint immobile. When combinations of devices are used on the same vertebral joint, the device value coded for the procedure is as follows:

- If an interbody fusion device is used to render the joint immobile (alone or containing other material like bone graft), the procedure is coded with the device value Interbody Fusion Device.
- If internal fixation is used to render the joint immobile and an interbody fusion device is not used, the procedure is coded with the device value Internal Fixation Device.
- If bone graft is the only device used to render the joint immobile, the procedure is coded with the device value Nonautologous Tissue Substitute or Autologous Tissue Substitute.
- If a mixture of autologous and nonautologous bone graft (with or without biological or synthetic extenders or binders) is used to render the joint immobile, code the procedure with the device value Autologous Tissue Substitute.

Examples: Fusion of a vertebral joint using a cage style interbody fusion device containing morsellized bone graft is coded to the device Interbody Fusion Device.
Fusion of a vertebral joint using a bone dowel interbody fusion device made of cadaver bone and packed with a mixture of local morsellized bone and demineralized bone matrix is coded to the device Interbody Fusion Device.
Fusion of a vertebral joint using rigid plates affixed with screws and reinforced with bone cement is coded to the device Internal Fixation Device.
Fusion of a vertebral joint using both autologous bone graft and bone bank bone graft is coded to the device Autologous Tissue Substitute.

Inspection Procedures

B3.11a. Inspection of a body part(s) performed in order to achieve the objective of a procedure is not coded separately.

Example: Fiberoptic bronchoscopy performed for irrigation of bronchus, only the irrigation procedure is coded.

B3.11b. If multiple tubular body parts are inspected, the most distal body part inspected is coded. If multiple non-tubular body parts in a region are inspected, the body part that specifies the entire area inspected is coded.

Examples: Cystoureteroscopy with inspection of bladder and ureters is coded to the ureter body part value.
Exploratory laparotomy with general inspection of abdominal contents is coded to the peritoneal cavity body part value.

B3.11c. When both an Inspection procedure and another procedure are performed on the same body part during the same episode, if the

Inspection procedure is performed using a different approach than the other procedure, the Inspection procedure is coded separately.
Example: Endoscopic Inspection of the duodenum is coded separately when open Excision of the duodenum is performed during the same procedural episode.

Occlusion vs. Restriction for Vessel Embolization Procedures
B3.12. If the objective of an embolization procedure is to completely close a vessel, the root operation Occlusion is coded. If the objective of an embolization procedure is to narrow the lumen of a vessel, the root operation Restriction is coded.

Examples: Tumor embolization is coded to the root operation Occlusion, because the objective of the procedure is to cut off the blood supply to the vessel.
Embolization of a cerebral aneurysm is coded to the root operation Restriction, because the objective of the procedure is not to close off the vessel entirely, but to narrow the lumen of the vessel at the site of the aneurysm where it is abnormally wide.

Release Procedures
B3.13. In the root operation Release, the body part value coded is the body part being freed and not the tissue being manipulated or cut to free the body part.

Example: Lysis of intestinal adhesions is coded to the specific intestine body part value.

Release vs. Division
B3.14. If the sole objective of the procedure is freeing a body part without cutting the body part, the root operation is Release. If the sole objective of the procedure is separating or transecting a body part, the root operation is Division.

Examples: Freeing a nerve root from surrounding scar tissue to relieve pain is coded to the root operation Release. Severing a nerve root to relieve pain is coded to the root operation Division.

Reposition for Fracture Treatment
B3.15. Reduction of a displaced fracture is coded to the root operation Reposition and the application of a cast or splint in conjunction with the Reposition procedure is not coded separately. Treatment of a nondisplaced fracture is coded to the procedure performed.

Examples: Putting a pin in a nondisplaced fracture is coded to the root operation Insertion.
Casting of a nondisplaced fracture is coded to the root operation Immobilization in the Placement section.

Transplantation vs. Administration

B3.16. Putting in a mature and functioning living body part taken from another individual or animal is coded to the root operation Transplantation. Putting in autologous or nonautologous cells is coded to the Administration section.

Example: Putting in autologous or nonautologous bone marrow, pancreatic islet cells or stem cells is coded to the Administration section.

B4. Body Part Guidelines

General Guidelines

B4.1a. If a procedure is performed on a portion of a body part that does not have a separate body part value, code the body part value corresponding to the whole body part.

Example: A procedure performed on the alveolar process of the mandible is coded to the mandible body part.

B4.1b. If the prefix "peri" is used with a body part to identify the site of the procedure, the body part value is defined as the body part named.

Example: A procedure site identified as perirenal is coded to the kidney body part.

Branches of Body Parts

B4.2. Where a specific branch of a body part does not have its own body part value in PCS, the body part is coded to the closest proximal branch that has a specific body part value.

Example: A procedure performed on the mandibular branch of the trigeminal nerve is coded to the trigeminal nerve body part value

Bilateral Body Part Values

B4.3. Bilateral body part values are available for a limited number of body parts. If the identical procedure is performed on contralateral body parts, and a bilateral body part value exists for that body part, a single procedure is coded using the bilateral body part value. If no bilateral body part value exists, each procedure is coded separately using the appropriate body part value.

Example: The identical procedure performed on both fallopian tubes is coded once using the body part value Fallopian Tube, Bilateral. The identical procedure performed on both knee joints is coded twice using the body part values Knee Joint, Right and Knee Joint, Left.

Coronary Arteries

B4.4. The coronary arteries are classified as a single body part that is further specified by number of sites treated and not by name or number of arteries. Separate body part values are used to specify the number of sites treated when the same procedure is performed on multiple sites in the coronary arteries.

Examples: Angioplasty of two distinct sites in the left anterior descending coronary artery with placement of two stents is coded as Dilation of Coronary Arteries, Two Sites, with Intraluminal Device. Angioplasty of two distinct sites in the left anterior descending coronary artery, one with stent placed and one without, is coded separately as Dilation of Coronary Artery, One Site with Intraluminal Device, and Dilation of Coronary Artery, One Site with no device.

Tendons, Ligaments, Bursae and Fascia near a Joint

B4.5. Procedures performed on tendons, ligaments, bursae and fascia supporting a joint are coded to the body part in the respective body system that is the focus of the procedure. Procedures performed on joint structures themselves are coded to the body part in the joint body systems.

Example: Repair of the anterior cruciate ligament of the knee is coded to the knee bursae and ligament body part in the bursae and ligaments body system. Knee arthroscopy with shaving of articular cartilage is coded to the knee joint body part in the Lower Joints body system.

Skin, Subcutaneous Tissue and Fascia Overlying a Joint

B4.6. If a procedure is performed on the skin, subcutaneous tissue or fascia overlying a joint, the procedure is coded to the following body part:

- Shoulder is coded to Upper Arm
- Elbow is coded to Lower Arm
- Wrist is coded to Lower Arm
- Hip is coded to Upper Leg
- Knee is coded to Lower Leg
- Ankle is coded to Foot

Fingers and Toes

B4.7 If a body system does not contain a separate body part value for fingers, procedures performed on the fingers are coded to the body part value for the hand. If a body system does not contain a separate body part value for toes, procedures performed on the toes are coded to the body part value for the foot.

Example: Excision of finger muscle is coded to one of the hand muscle body part values in the Muscles body system.

B5. Approach Guidelines

B5.2. Procedures performed using the open approach with percutaneous endoscopic assistance are coded to the approach Open.

Example: Laparoscopic-assisted sigmoidectomy is coded to the approach Open.

External Approach

B5.3a. Procedures performed within an orifice on structures that are visible without the aid of any instrumentation are coded to the approach External.

Example: Resection of tonsils is coded to the approach External.

B5.3b. Procedures performed indirectly by the application of external force through the intervening body layers are coded to the approach External.

Example: Closed reduction of fracture is coded to the approach External.

Percutaneous Procedure via Device

B5.4. Procedures performed percutaneously via a device placed for the procedure are coded to the approach Percutaneous.

Example: Fragmentation of kidney stone performed via percutaneous nephrostomy is coded to the approach Percutaneous.

B6. Device Guidelines

General Guidelines

B6.1a. A device is coded only if a device remains after the procedure is completed. If no device remains, the device value No Device is coded.

B6.1b. Materials such as sutures, ligatures, radiological markers and temporary post-operative wound drains are considered integral to the performance of a procedure and are not coded as devices.

B6.1c. Procedures performed on a device only and not on a body part are specified in the root operations Change, Irrigation, Removal and Revision, and are coded to the procedure performed.

Example: Irrigation of percutaneous nephrostomy tube is coded to the root operation Irrigation of indwelling device in the Administration section.

Drainage Device

B6.2. A separate procedure to put in a drainage device is coded to the root operation Drainage with the device value Drainage Device.

Obstetric Section Guidelines (Section 1)

Products of Conception

C1. Procedures performed on the products of conception are coded to the Obstetrics section. Procedures performed on the pregnant female other than the products of conception are coded to the appropriate root operation in the Medical and Surgical section.

Example: Amniocentesis is coded to the products of conception body part in the Obstetrics section. Repair of obstetric urethral laceration is coded to the urethra body part in the Medical and Surgical section.

Procedures Following Delivery or Abortion

C2. Procedures performed following a delivery or abortion for curettage of the endometrium or evacuation of retained products of conception are all coded in the Obstetrics section, to the root operation Extraction and the body part Products of Conception, Retained. Diagnostic or therapeutic dilation and curettage performed during times other than the postpartum or post-abortion period are all coded in the Medical and Surgical section, to the root operation Extraction and the body part Endometrium.

Source: CMS 2011b

Activity 10: ICD-10-PCS Coding Guidelines

Select the guidelines to code the following procedure.

1. Laparoscopic cholecystectomy converted to an open cholecystectomy
   a. Diagnostic excision
   b. Approach
   c. Device
   d. Discontinued procedure
   e. Multiple procedures

2. Biopsy of breast followed by partial mastectomy at the same operative site
   a. Diagnostic excision
   b. Approach
   c. Device
   d. Inspection
   e. Multiple procedures

3. Total excision of right lobe of liver
   a. Diagnostic excision
   b. Approach
   c. Device
   d. Excision vs. Resection
   e. Multiple procedures

4. Closed reduction of fracture
   a. Diagnostic excision
   b. Approach
   c. Device
   d. Control
   e. Multiple procedures

5. Coronary bypass with excision of saphenous vein graft
   a. Diagnostic excision
   b. Approach
   c. Device
   d. Inspection
   e. Multiple procedures

Documentation Guidelines

General Documentation Guidelines

The clinical detail found in many ICD-10-PCS codes is greater or, in some cases, different than that currently found in ICD-9-CM. In order to code in ICD-10-PCS, you will need to consider these differences.

Example:

- The "Omit code" is found in the Index of ICD-9-CM Volume 3. This means procedures performed only for the purpose of performing further surgery, namely, incisions, or those that represent operative approach are not coded.
- However, in the case of ICD-10-PCS, approach is one of the seven components that comprise a code from the Medical and Surgical section.

Note: Physician education on the various aspects of procedure classification will be necessary in order to code to the highest level of specificity in ICD-10-PCS. For example, note the additional detail in the following ICD-10-PCS codes in comparison to ICD-9-CM Volume 3 codes.

Section-Specific Documentation Guidelines

In preparation for implementation of ICD-10-PCS, coding professionals should examine the most commonly assigned procedures in each ICD-10-PCS section and determine the necessary clinician education. Identifying where documentation improvement is needed most and focusing training in those areas will help ease the transition to the new system.

To provide a starting point for this education, a couple of examples from each ICD-10-PCS section have been selected for review and analysis. Take a look at each pair, compare the descriptions, and note what must be documented to support the ICD-10-PCS code assignment.

Medical and Surgical Section – Example 1			
ICD-10-PCS	**Description**	**ICD-9-CM**	**Description**
0V508ZZ	Transurethral endoscopic laser ablation of prostate	60.21	Transurethral guided laser induced prostatectomy

Medical and Surgical Section – Example 2			
ICD-10-PCS	**Description**	**ICD-9-CM**	**Description**
0MN14ZZ	Right shoulder arthroscopy with coracoacromial ligament release	80.41	Release of ligament, shoulder

Medical and Surgical-related Section – Example 1			
ICD-10-PCS	**Description**	**ICD-9-CM**	**Description**
3E0P7LZ	Transvaginal artificial insemination	69.92	Artificial insemination

Medical and Surgical-related Section – Example 2			
ICD-10-PCS	**Description**	**ICD-9-CM**	**Description**
5A1945Z	Continuous mechanical ventilation, 40 consecutive hours	96.71	Continuous mechanical ventilation for less than 96 consecutive hours

Ancillary Section – Example 1			
ICD-10-PCS	**Description**	**ICD-9-CM**	**Description**
BP04ZZZ	Portable x-ray of right clavicle, limited study	87.43	X-ray of ribs, sternum, and clavicle

Ancillary Section – Example 2			
ICD-10-PCS	**Description**	**ICD-9-CM**	**Description**
GZB1ZZZ	ECT (electroconvulsive therapy), unilateral multiple seizure	94.27	Other electroshock therapy

Section 6 Review Questions

1. True or False? If an intended procedure is discontinued, no code is assigned.
   a. True
   b. False

2. Which of the following guidelines would you use when coding fiberoptic bronchoscopy with irrigation of bronchus?
   a. Guideline B3.2c: During the same operative episode, multiple procedures are coded if multiple root operations with distinct objectives are performed on the same body part
   b. Guideline B3.11a: Inspection of a body part(s) performed in order to achieve the objective of a procedure is not coded separately
   c. Guideline B3.2a: During the same operative episode, multiple procedures are coded if the same root operation is performed on different body parts as defined by distinct values of the body part character
   d. Guideline B3.4: If a diagnostic excision, extraction, or drainage procedure (biopsy) is followed by a more definitive procedure, such as destruction, excision, or resection at the same procedure site, both the biopsy and the more definitive treatment are coded

3. What would you need to look for in the documentation if you were coding in ICD-10-PCS rather than ICD-9-CM Volume 3 for the following procedure: Cryotherapy of wart on left hand
   a. The site, skin
   b. The site, left hand
   c. The root operation, destruction
   d. The diagnosis, wart

Final Review Questions

1. Which of the following characteristic was *not* identified as essential in the development of ICD-10-PCS?
   a. Expandability
   b. Completeness
   c. Single axis
   d. Standard terminology

2. ICD-10-PCS codes are ____________.
   a. Three to four digits long with a decimal point placed after the second digit
   b. Six characters long
   c. Six characters long with a decimal point after the third digit
   d. Seven characters long

3. True or False? All ICD-10-PCS alphanumeric codes begin with an alpha character.
   a. True
   b. False

4. What are the seven spaces of an ICD-10-PCS code called?
   a. Values
   b. Characters
   c. Sections
   d. Qualifiers

5. Which value represents an Ancillary section in ICD-10-PCS?
   a. Section value 1
   b. Section value D
   c. Section value 0
   d. Section value E

6. Root operation tables within the Medical and Surgical section (first character 0) consist of ____________.
   a. Three columns and a single row
   b. Three columns and a varying number of rows
   c. Four columns and a single row
   d. Four columns and a varying number of rows

7. True or False? A combination of characters not in a single row of a Table is *not* a valid code.
   a. True
   b. False

8. Which of the following codes is found in the Medical and Surgical-related section, Obstetrics, of ICD-10-PCS?
   a. 2W20X4Z
   b. 10E0XZZ
   c. 3E1U38Z
   d. BW03ZZZ

9. True or False? For the Medical and Surgical section, main terms in the Index are based on the third character value.
   a. True
   b. False

10. True or False? One characteristic of the key attribute "completeness" is each code retains its unique definition.
   a. True
   b. False

11. Which of the following ICD-10-PCS characteristics addresses the problematic ICD-9-CM code 28.11, Biopsy of tonsils and adenoids?
   a. Diagnosis information excluded
   b. Standardized terminology
   c. NOS code options excluded
   d. Limited NEC code options

12. Which of the following procedures would be classified to the root operation Resection?
   a. Total mastectomy
   b. Breast lumpectomy
   c. Suction dilation and curettage
   d. Fulguration of endometrium

13. Which of the following is the correct definition for a "percutaneous endoscopic" approach?
   a. Entry, by puncture or minor incision, of instrumentation through the skin or mucous membrane and/or any other body layer necessary to reach the site of the procedure
   b. Cutting through the skin or mucous membrane and any other body layers necessary to expose the site of the procedure, and entry, by puncture or minor incision, of instrumentation through the skin or mucous membrane and any other body layers necessary to aid in the performance of the procedure
   c. Entry, by puncture or minor incision, of instrumentation through the skin or mucous membrane and/or any other body layers necessary to reach and visualize the site of the procedure
   d. Entry of instrumentation through a natural or artificial opening to reach and visualize the site of the procedure

14. Which of the following is an example of a qualifier?
    a. Excision
    b. Orthopedic pins
    c. Diagnostic
    d. Resection

15. Correcting, to the extent possible, a malfunctioning or displaced device is the definition of ___________.
    a. Replacement
    b. Revision
    c. Resection
    d. Release

16. True or False? The following diagram represents the organizational structure of the Medical and Surgical section.

Character 1 Section	Character 2 Body System	Character 3 Root Operation	Character 4 Body System	Character 5 Approach	Character 6 Substance	Character 7 Qualifier

    a. True
    b. False

17. Which of the following procedures is assigned to the Medical and Surgical-related sections of ICD-10-PCS?
    a. Percutaneous ligation of esophageal vein
    b. PTA of right brachial artery stenosis
    c. Placement of intrathecal infusion pump for pain management, percutaneous
    d. Epidural injection of mixed steroid and local anesthetic for pain control

18. True or False? The following diagram represents the organizational structure of the Obstetrics section found in the Medical and Surgical-related sections.

Character 1 Section	Character 2 Body System	Character 3 Root Operation	Character 4 Body Part	Character 5 Approach	Character 6 Device	Character 7 Qualifier

    a. True
    b. False

19. Which of the following is *not* one of the Ancillary sections?
    a. Radiation Oncology
    b. Nuclear Medicine
    c. Mental Health
    d. Obstetrics

20. True or False? During the same operative episode, multiple procedures are coded if multiple root operations with distinct objectives are performed on the same body part.
    a. True
    b. False

Part I: ICD-10-PCS Coding

ICD-10-PCS Training – Day 1

ICD-10-PCS Resources – References

2011 ICD-10-PCS available at www.cms.hhs.gov/ICD10

- **2011 Code Tables and Index**
    - ICD-10-PCS 2011 Tables
    - Definitions
    - Index
- ***2011 ICD-10-PCS Reference Manual***
    - Chapter 1: ICD-10-PCS Overview
    - Chapter 2: Procedures in the Medical and Surgical Section
    - Chapter 3: Procedures in the Medical and Surgical-related Sections
    - Chapter 4: Procedures in the Ancillary Sections
    - Appendix A: ICD-10-PCS Definitions
    - Appendix B: ICD-10-PCS Draft Coding Guidelines
        - Conventions
        - Medical and Surgical Section (Section 0)
        - Obstetrics Section Guidelines (Section 1)
- 2011 ICD-10-PCS Slides
    - PCS 2011 Slides – PowerPoint Presentation
- 2011 Official ICD-10-PCS Coding Guidelines
- 2011 Development of the ICD-10 Procedure Coding System
- 2011 Version – What's New
- 2011 Mapping "ICD-10-PCS to ICD-9-CM" and "ICD-9-CM to ICD-10-PCS"; and User Guide, Reimbursement Guide, Procedures
- 2011 Code Descriptions
- 2011 Addendum

ICD-10-PCS: The Complete Official Draft Code Set 2011 Ingenix (referred to throughout this manual as the *ICD-10-PCS 2011 Code Book*)

- Introduction (1–17)
- ICD-10-PCS Draft Coding Guidelines (19–23)
- Index (33–125)
- ICD-10-PCS Tables by Body System and Section (127–481)
- Appendix A: Root Operations Definitions (483–488)
- Appendix B: Comparison of Medical and Surgical Root Operations (489–491)
- Appendix C: Body Part Key (493–512)
- Appendix D: Type and Type Qualifier Definitions Sections B-H (513–522)
- Appendix E: Components of the Medical and Surgical Approach Definitions (523)
- Appendix F: Character Meanings (525–583)

Discussion of ICD-10-PCS Definitions and Guidelines

Guidelines

The ICD-10-PCS Draft Coding Guidelines (2011) are included in the *ICD-10-PCS 2011 Code Book*. There are three main sections of guidelines:

A. Conventions
B. Medical and Surgical Section (section 0)
C. Obstetrics Section Guidelines (section 1)

Section B is by far the most extensive section. There are guidelines for:

- Body System
- Root Operation
- Body Part
- Approach
- Device

An effort has been made to incorporate the various guidelines into the learning content of this training, but some of the guidelines have overarching principals that must be understood before proceeding.

Conventions

A1. ICD-10-PCS codes are composed of seven characters. Each character is an axis of classification that specifies information about the procedure performed. Within a defined code range, a character specifies the same type of information in that axis of classification.

Example: The fifth axis of classification specifies the approach in sections 0 through 4 and 7 through 9 of the system.

A2. One of 34 possible values can be assigned to each axis of classification in the seven-character code: they are the numbers 0 through 9 and the alphabet (except [the letters] I and O because they are easily confused with the numbers 1 and 0). The number of unique values used in an axis of classification differs as needed.

Example: Where the fifth axis of classification specifies the approach, seven different approach values are currently used to specify the approach.

A3. The valid values for an axis of classification can be added to as needed.

Example: If a significantly distinct type of device is used in a new procedure, a new device value can be added to the system.

A4. As with words in their context, the meaning of any single value is a combination of its axis of classification and any preceding values on which it may be dependent.

Example: The meaning of a body part value in the Medical and Surgical section is always dependent on the body system value. The body part value 0 in the Central

Nervous body system specifies Brain and the body part value 0 in the Peripheral Nervous body system specifies Cervical Plexus.

A5. As the system is expanded to become increasingly detailed, over time more values will depend on preceding values for their meaning.

Example: In the Lower Joints body system, the device value 3 in the root operation Insertion specifies Infusion Device and the device value 3 in the root operation Fusion specifies Interbody Fusion Device.

A6. The purpose of the Alphabetic Index is to locate the appropriate table that contains all information necessary to construct a procedure code. The PCS Tables should always be consulted to find the most appropriate valid code.

A7. It is not required to consult the index first before proceeding to the tables to complete the code. A valid code may be chosen directly from the tables.

A8. All seven characters must be specified to be a valid code. If the documentation is incomplete for coding purposes, the physician should be queried for the necessary information.

A9. Within a PCS table, valid codes include all combinations of choices in characters 4 through 7 contained in the same row of the table. In the following example, 0JHT3VZ is a valid code, and 0JHW3VZ is *not* a valid code.

Section: **0: Medical and Surgical**
Body System: **J: Subcutaneous Tissue and Fascia**
Operation: **H: Insertion:** Putting in a nonbiological appliance that monitors, assists, performs, or prevents a physiological function but does not physically take the place of a body part.

Body Part	Approach	Device	Qualifier
S Subcutaneous Tissue and Fascia, Head and Neck **V** Subcutaneous Tissue and Fascia, Upper Extremity **W** Subcutaneous Tissue and Fascia, Lower Extremity	**0** Open **3** Percutaneous	**1** Radioactive Element **3** Infusion Device	**Z** No Qualifier
T Subcutaneous Tissue and Fascia, Trunk	**0** Open **3** Percutaneous	**1** Radioactive Element **3** Infusion Device **V** Infusion Pump	**Z** No Qualifier

A10. "And," when used in a code description, means "and/or."

Example: Lower Arm and Wrist Muscle means lower arm and/or wrist muscle.

A11. Many of the terms used to construct PCS codes are defined within the system. It is the coder's responsibility to determine what the documentation in the medical record equates to in the PCS definitions. The physician is not expected to use the terms used in PCS code descriptions, nor is the coder required to query the physician when the correlation between the documentation and the defined PCS terms is clear.

Example: When the physician documents "partial resection," the coder can independently correlate "partial resection" to the root operation Excision without querying the physician for clarification.

Coding Note: Main index term is a root operation, root procedure type, or common procedure name. Examples are:

- Resection (root operation)
- Fluoroscopy (root type)
- Prostatectomy (common procedure name)

Coding Note: When reviewing tables, sometimes there are multiple tables for the first three characters and they may cover multiple pages in the code book.

Discussion of ICD-10-PCS Definitions and Guidelines in the Medical and Surgical Section – Section 0

ICD-10-PCS Section

All codes in ICD-10-PCS are seven characters. The letters O and I are not used in PCS so as not to be confused with the numbers 0 and 1. Each character has a meaning and the meanings change by sections, or the broad procedure category.

The section provides the first character value. The sections of ICD-10-PCS are:

Section Value	Description
0	Medical and Surgical
1	Obstetrics
2	Placement
3	Administration
4	Measurement and Monitoring
5	Extracorporeal Assistance and Performance
6	Extracorporeal Therapies
7	Osteopathic
8	Other Procedures
9	Chiropractic
B	Imaging
C	Nuclear Medicine
D	Radiation Oncology
F	Physical Rehabilitation and Diagnostic Audiology
G	Mental Health
H	Substance Abuse Treatment

ICD-10-PCS Body System

The second character defines the body system, or the general physiological system or anatomical region involved. This way of categorizing into larger groupings makes the tables easier to navigate and also provides information quickly about the procedure. All procedures with the same second character would be of the same anatomical region or system.

Medical and Surgical Section Body Systems

Body System	Value	Body System	Value
Central Nervous (525)	0	Subcutaneous Tissue and Fascia (541)	J
Peripheral Nervous (526)	1	Muscles (542)	K
Heart and Great Vessels (527)	2	Tendons – Includes synovial membrane (543)	L
Upper Arteries (528)	3	Bursae and Ligaments – Includes synovial membrane (544)	M
Lower Arteries (529)	4	Head and Facial Bones (545)	N
Upper Veins (530)	5	Upper Bones (546)	P
Lower Veins (531)	6	Lower Bones (547)	Q
Lymphatic and Hemic – Includes lymph vessels and lymph nodes (532)	7	Upper Joints – Includes synovial membrane (548)	R
Eye (533)	8	Lower Joints – Includes synovial membrane (549)	S
Ear, Nose, Sinus – Includes sinus ducts (534)	9	Urinary (550)	T
Respiratory (535)	B	Female Reproductive (551)	U
Mouth and Throat (536)	C	Male Reproductive (552)	V
Gastrointestinal (537)	D	Anatomical Regions, General (553)	W
Hepatobiliary and Pancreas (538)	F	Anatomical Regions, Upper Extremities (554)	X
Endocrine (539)	G	Anatomical Regions, Lower Extremities (555)	Y
Skin and Breast – Includes skin and breast glands and ducts (540)	H		

Note: In the *ICD-10-PCS 2011 Code Book*, Appendix F lists the Character Meanings available by Body Systems. These page numbers are listed in the preceding table for easy reference.

Body System Guidelines

General Guidelines

B2.1a. The procedure codes in the general anatomical regions body systems should only be used when the procedure is performed on an anatomical region rather than a specific body part (for example, root operations Control and

Detachment, drainage of a body cavity) or on the rare occasion when no information is available to support assignment of a code to a specific body part.

Example: Control of postoperative hemorrhage is coded to the root operation Control found in the general anatomical regions body systems.

B2.1b. Body systems designated as upper or lower contain body parts located above or below the diaphragm, respectively.

Example: Vein body parts above the diaphragm are found in the Upper Veins body system; vein body parts below the diaphragm are found in the Lower Veins body system.

ICD-10-PCS Root Operations

The third character defines the root operation, or the **objective** of the procedure. There are 31 root operations, and they are arranged by groups with similar attributes. If multiple procedures as defined by distinct objectives are performed, multiple codes are assigned.

Examples of root operations are:

- Bypass
- Drainage
- Reattachment
- Resection
- Inspection

Refer to *ICD-10-PCS 2011 Code Book* Appendix A (pages 483–485). Note: Pages 485–488 refer to sections other than the Medical and Surgical Section. Appendix B includes a comparison of the Medical and Surgical Root Operations.

List of Root Operations for the Medical and Surgical Section

Medical and Surgical Section Root Operations			
Alteration	Division	Inspection	Reposition
Bypass	Drainage	Map	Resection
Change	Excision	Occlusion	Restriction
Control	Extirpation	Reattachment	Revision
Creation	Extraction	Release	Supplement
Destruction	Fragmentation	Removal	Transfer
Detachment	Fusion	Repair	Transplantation
Dilation	Insertion	Replacement	

Root Operation Guidelines

General Guidelines

B3.1a. In order to determine the appropriate root operation, the full definition of the root operation, as contained in the PCS Tables, must be applied.

B3.1b. Components of a procedure specified in the root operation definition and explanation are not coded separately. Procedural steps necessary to reach the operative site and close the operative site are also not coded separately.

Example: Resection of a joint as part of a joint replacement procedure is included in the root operation definition of Replacement and is not coded separately. Laparotomy performed to reach the site of an open liver biopsy is not coded separately.

Multiple Procedures

B3.2. During the same operative episode, multiple procedures are coded if:

a. The same root operation is performed on different body parts as defined by distinct values of the body part character.

   Example: Diagnostic excision of liver and pancreas are coded separately.

b. The same root operation is repeated at different body sites that are included in the same body part value.

   Example: Excision of the sartorius muscle and excision of the gracilis muscle are both included in the upper leg muscle body part value, and multiple procedures are coded.

c. Multiple root operations with distinct objectives are performed on the same body part.

   Example: Destruction of sigmoid lesion and bypass of sigmoid colon are coded separately.

d. The intended root operation is attempted using one approach, but is converted to a different approach.

   Example: Laparoscopic cholecystectomy converted to an open cholecystectomy is coded as percutaneous endoscopic Inspection and open Resection.

Discontinued Procedures

B3.3. If the intended procedure is discontinued, code the procedure to the root operation performed. If a procedure is discontinued before any other root operation is performed, code the root operation Inspection of the body part or anatomical region inspected.

Example: A planned aortic valve replacement procedure is discontinued after the initial thoracotomy and before any incision is made in the heart muscle, when the patient becomes hemodynamically unstable. This procedure is coded as an open Inspection of the mediastinum.

Biopsy Followed by more Definitive Treatment

B3.4. If a diagnostic Excision, Extraction, or Drainage procedure (biopsy) is followed by a more definitive procedure such as Destruction, Excision, or Resection at the same procedure site, both the biopsy and the more definitive treatment are coded.

Example: Biopsy of breast followed by partial mastectomy at the same procedure site, both the biopsy and the partial mastectomy procedure are coded.

Overlapping Body Layers

B3.5. If the root operations Excision, Repair, or Inspection are performed on overlapping layers of the musculoskeletal system, the body part specifying the deepest layer is coded.

Example: Excisional debridement that includes skin and subcutaneous tissue and muscle is coded to the muscle body part.

Coding Note: The specific Root Operation Guidelines (B3.6a–B 3.16) are presented in the appropriate section of training.

ICD-10-PCS Body Part

The fourth character defines the body part or specific anatomical site where the procedure was performed. This is the specific site, different from character 2 that provided the general body system. There are 34 possible body part values in each body system.

Examples of body parts are:

- Liver
- Kidney
- Thalamus
- Ascending Colon
- Optic Nerve
- Tonsil

Body Part Guidelines

B4.1a. If a procedure is performed on a portion of a body part that does not have a separate body part value, code the body part value corresponding to the whole body part.

Example: A procedure performed on the alveolar process of the mandible is coded to the mandible body part.

B4.1b. If the prefix "peri" is used with a body part to identify the site of the procedure, the body part value is defined as the body part named.

Example: A procedure site identified as perirenal is coded to the kidney body part.

Branches of Body Parts

B4.2. Where a specific branch of a body part does not have its own body part value in PCS, the body part is coded to the closest proximal branch that has a specific body part value.

Example: A procedure performed on the mandibular branch of the trigeminal nerve is coded to the trigeminal nerve body part value.

Bilateral Body Part Values

B4.3. Bilateral body part values are available for a limited number of body parts. If the identical procedure is performed on contralateral body parts, and a bilateral body part value exists for that body part, a single procedure is coded using the bilateral body part value. If no bilateral body part value exists, each procedure is coded separately using the appropriate body part value.

Example: The identical procedure performed on both fallopian tubes is coded once using the body part value Fallopian Tube, Bilateral. The identical procedure performed on both knee joints is coded twice using the body part values Knee Joint, Right and Knee Joint, Left.

Coronary Arteries

B4.4. The coronary arteries are classified as a single body part that is further specified by number of sites treated and not by name or number of arteries. Separate body part values are used to specify the number of sites treated when the same procedure is performed on multiple sites in the coronary arteries.

Examples:

- Angioplasty of two distinct sites in the left anterior descending coronary artery with placement of two stents is coded as Dilation of Coronary Arteries, Two Sites, with Intraluminal Device.
- Angioplasty of two distinct sites in the left anterior descending coronary artery, one with stent placed and one without, is coded separately as Dilation of Coronary Artery, One Site with Intraluminal Device, and Dilation of Coronary Artery, One Site with No Device.

Tendons, Ligaments, Bursae and Fascia Near a Joint

B4.5. Procedures performed on tendons, ligaments, bursae and fascia supporting a joint are coded to the body part in the respective body system that is the focus of the procedure. Procedures performed on joint structures themselves are coded to the body part in the joint body systems.

Example: Repair of the anterior cruciate ligament of the knee is coded to the knee bursae and ligament body part in the bursae and ligaments body system. Knee arthroscopy with shaving of articular cartilage is coded to the knee joint body part in the Lower Joints body system.

Skin, Subcutaneous Tissue and Fascia Overlying a Joint

B4.6. If a procedure is performed on the skin, subcutaneous tissue, or fascia overlying a joint, the procedure is coded to the following body part:

- Shoulder is coded to Upper Arm
- Elbow is coded to Lower Arm
- Wrist is coded to Lower Arm
- Hip is coded to Upper Leg
- Knee is coded to Lower Leg
- Ankle is coded to Foot

Fingers and Toes

B4.7. If a body system does not contain a separate body part value for fingers, procedures performed on the fingers are coded to the body part value for the hand. If a body system does not contain a separate body part value for toes, procedures performed on the toes are coded to the body part value for the foot.

Example: Excision of finger muscle is coded to one of the hand muscle body part values in the Muscles body system.

Coding Note: Central Nervous System (0) vs. Peripheral Nervous System (1)

- It is important to review anatomy regarding nerves (Appendix F, pages 525–526 of the *ICD-10-PCS 2011 Code Book* will be helpful.)
- Examples of Central Nervous System: brain, optic nerve, trigeminal nerve, vagus nerve, spinal meninges
- Examples of Peripheral Nervous System: cervical nerve, ulnar nerve, radial nerve, thoracic nerve, tibial nerve, sciatic nerve, sacral plexus

ICD-10-PCS Approaches

The fifth character defines the approach or the technique used to reach the procedure site. There are seven different approach values in the Medical and Surgical section.

Approaches may be through the skin or mucous membrane, through an orifice, or external.

Approaches through the skin or mucous membranes:

- Open
- Percutaneous
- Percutaneous Endoscopic

Approaches through an orifice:

- Via Natural or Artificial Opening
- Via Natural or Artificial Opening Endoscopic
- Via Natural or Artificial Opening With Percutaneous Endoscopic Assistance

Note: When assigning the approach value, remember that the approach defines the technique used to reach the procedure site, not necessarily the instruments used.

ICD-10-PCS Approaches

Value	Approach	Definition	Applicable Guidelines	Examples
0	**Open**	Cutting through the skin or mucous membrane and any other body layers necessary to expose the site of the procedure.	B5.2	Open CABG Open endarterectomy Open resection cecum Abdominal hysterectomy
3	**Percutaneous**	Entry, by puncture or minor incision, of instrumentation through the skin or mucous membrane and any other body layers necessary to reach the site of the procedure.	B5.4	Percutaneous needle core biopsy of kidney Liposuction Percutaneous drainage of ascites Needle biopsy of liver
4	**Percutaneous Endoscopic**	Entry, by puncture or minor incision, of instrumentation through the skin or mucous membrane and any other body layers necessary to reach and visualize the site of the procedure.		Laparoscopic cholecystectomy Laparoscopy with destruction of endometriosis Endoscopic drainage of sinus Arthroscopy
7	**Via Natural or Artificial Opening**	Entry of instrumentation through a natural or artificial external opening to reach the site of the procedure.		Foley catheter placement Transvaginal intraluminal cervical cerclage Digital rectal exam Endotracheal intubation
8	**Via Natural or Artificial Opening Endoscopic**	Entry of instrumentation through a natural or artificial external opening to reach and visualize the site of the procedure.		Transurethral cystoscopy with removal bladder stone Endoscopic ERCP Hysteroscopy Colonoscopy EGD Sigmoidoscopy
F	**Via Natural or Artificial Opening With Percutaneous Endoscopic Assistance**	Entry of instrumentation through a natural or artificial external opening and entry, by puncture or minor incision, of instrumentation through the skin or mucous membrane and any other body layers necessary to aid in the performance of the procedure.		Laparoscopic-assisted vaginal hysterectomy (LAVH)
X	**External**	Procedures performed directly on the skin or mucous membrane and procedures performed indirectly by the application of external force through the skin or mucous membrane.	B5.3a B5.3b	Resection of tonsils Closed reduction of fracture Excision of skin lesion Cautery nosebleed Manual rupture joint adhesions Reattachment severed ear

For additional information, refer to the *ICD-10-PCS 2011 Code Book* (page 523 of Appendix E).

Approach Guidelines

Open Approach with Percutaneous Endoscopic Assistance

B5.2. Procedures performed using the open approach with percutaneous endoscopic assistance are coded to the approach Open.

Example: Laparoscopic-assisted sigmoidectomy is coded to the approach Open.

External Approach

B5.3a. Procedures performed within an orifice on structures that are visible without the aid of any instrumentation are coded to the approach External.

Example: Resection of tonsils is coded to the approach External.

B5.3b. Procedures performed indirectly by the application of external force through the intervening body layers are coded to the approach External.

Example: Closed reduction of fracture is coded to the approach External.

Percutaneous Procedure via Device

B5.4. Procedures performed percutaneously via a device placed for the procedure are coded to the approach Percutaneous.

Example: Fragmentation of kidney stone performed via percutaneous nephrostomy is coded to the approach Percutaneous.

ICD-10-PCS Device

There may be a device left in place, depending on the procedure performed. The sixth character identifies these devices. Device values fall into four basic groups:

- Grafts and Prostheses
- Implants
- Simple or Mechanical Appliances
- Electronic Appliances

The four general types of devices are:

- Biological or synthetic material that takes the place of all or a portion of a body part (for example, skin graft, joint prosthesis).
- Biological or synthetic material that assists or prevents a physiological function (for example, urinary catheter, IUD).
- Therapeutic material that is not absorbed by, eliminated by, or incorporated into a body part (for example, radioactive implant). Therapeutic materials that are considered devices can be removed.
- Mechanical or electronic appliances used to assist, monitor, take the place of, or prevent a physiological function (for example, diaphragmatic pacemaker, hearing device, cardiac pacemaker, orthopedic pins).

Coding Note: Devices
Only procedures that have a device that remains after the procedure is completed will have a specific device value assigned. Remember that all codes require seven characters. The default value to indicate that *no* device was involved is **Z**.

Examples of device values:

- Drainage device
- Radioactive element
- Autologous tissue substitute
- Extraluminal device
- Intraluminal device
- Synthetic substitute
- Nonautologous tissue substitute

In the Medical and Surgical section, two significant "not elsewhere classified" options are the root operation value Q, Repair and the device value Y, Other Device. Other Device is intended to be used to temporarily define new devices that do not have a specific value assigned, until one can be added to the system. No categories of medical or surgical devices are permanently classified to Other Device.

Coding Note: Materials incidental to a procedure such as clips and sutures are not considered devices.

Device Guidelines

General Guidelines

B6.1a. A device is coded only if a device remains after the procedure is completed. If no device remains, the device value No Device is coded.

B6.1b. Materials such as sutures, ligatures, radiological markers and temporary postoperative wound drains are considered integral to the performance of a procedure and are not coded as devices.

B6.1c. Procedures performed on a device only and not on a body part are specified in the root operations Change, Irrigation, Removal and Revision, and are coded to the procedure performed.

Example: Irrigation of percutaneous nephrostomy tube is coded to the root operation Irrigation of indwelling device in the Administration section.

Drainage Device

B6.2. A separate procedure to put in a drainage device is coded to the root operation Drainage with the device value Drainage Device.

ICD-10-PCS Qualifier

The seventh character defines a qualifier for the code that provides additional information about a specific attribute of the procedure. These qualifiers may have a narrow application, to a specific root operation, body system, or body part. There are no specific guidelines for qualifiers.

Examples of qualifiers:

- Type of transplant
- Second site for a bypass
- Diagnostic excision (biopsy)

> **Coding Note: Qualifiers**
> Most procedures will not have an applicable qualifier. The default value to indicate that *no* qualifier is needed is **Z**.

Device

Root Op

Y other Device

Valve Q

ICD-10-PCS Guidelines and Root Operations Review

ICD-10-PCS Guidelines

1. True or false? A biological or synthetic material that takes the place of all or a portion of a body part such as a joint prosthesis would qualify as a device in ICD-10-PCS.
   a. True
   b. False

2. True or false? According to ICD-10-PCS coding guidelines, if a diagnostic biopsy is followed by a therapeutic definitive procedure at the same site, code only the therapeutic excision or resection.
   a. True
   b. False

3. True or false? When coding in ICD-10-PCS, it is necessary to consult the Alphabetic Index and then proceed to the tables.
   a. True
   b. False

4. True or false? Lower arm and wrist muscle means lower arm and wrist muscle according to the definition of "and."
   a. True
   b. False

5. True or false? In the root operation, Release, the body part character is defined as the body part being freed and not the tissue that is being cut to free the body part.
   a. True
   b. False

6. True or false? Two codes would be assigned for this procedure: Resection of a joint with joint replacement.
   a. True
   b. False

7. True or false? If the prefix "peri" is used with a body part to identify the site of the procedure, the procedure is coded to the body part named.
   a. True
   b. False

8. True or false? Materials such as sutures, ligatures, radiological markers and temporary postop wound drains should be coded separately using ICD-10-PCS device codes.
   a. True
   b. False

9. True or false? Irrigation of a percutaneous nephrostomy tube is coded to the root operation Irrigation of indwelling device in the Administration section.
   a. True
   b. False

10. True or false? Body systems designated as upper or lower contain the body parts that are above or below the diaphragm respectively.
   a. True
   b. False

Root Operations

11. True or false? In ICD-10-PCS, when an entire lymph node chain is cut out, the appropriate root operation is Resection.
   a. True
   b. False

12. True or false? The root operation Detachment is used exclusively for amputation procedures.
   a. True
   b. False

13. True or false? Forceps removal of a foreign body is an example of an extirpation procedure.
   a. True
   b. False

release

14. True or false? The root operation Division is coded when the objective is to cut or separate the area around a body part, the attachments to a body part, or between subdivisions of a body that are causing abnormal constraint.
   a. True
   b. False

15. True or false? Adhesiolysis is an example of a release procedure.
   a. True
   b. False

16. True or false? The root operation Restriction is coded when the objective of the procedure is to close off a tubular body part or orifice.
   a. True
   b. False

17. True or false? The root operation Dilation is coded when the objective of the procedure is to enlarge the diameter of a tubular body part or orifice.
   a. True
   b. False

18. True or false? Typical Change procedures include exchange of drainage devices and feeding devices.
   a. True
   b. False

19. True or false? All codes in the ICD-10-PCS Administration section define procedures where a diagnostic or therapeutic substance is given to the patient, such as a platelet transfusion.
    a. True
    b. False

20. True or false? In ICD-10-PCS, the term *measurement* refers to a series of levels obtained at intervals, while *monitoring* describes a single level taken.
    a. True
    b. False

Coding Procedures in the Medical and Surgical Section – Section 0

The seven characters in the Medical and Surgical section are:

Susie buys Root Beer at Dairy Queen

Character 1 Section	Character 2 Body System	Character 3 Root Operation	Character 4 Body Part	Character 5 Approach	Character 6 Device	Character 7 Qualifier

1. Character 1 refers to the broad procedure category where the code is found (0) for Medical and Surgical.
2. Character 2 defines the body system or general physiological system or anatomical region.
3. Character 3 defines the root operation, or the objective of the procedure.
4. Character 4 defines the body part or anatomical site where the procedure was performed.
5. Character 5 defines the approach, or the technique used to reach the procedure site.
6. Character 6 defines the device (if any) left in place at the end of the procedure.
7. Character 7 defines the qualifier for the code.

Root Operation Groupings

There are nine groups of root operations, arranged by similar attributes:

- Root Operations That Take Out Some or All of a Body Part
- Root Operations That Take Out Solids/ Fluids/Gases From a Body Part
- Root Operations Involving Cutting or Separation Only
- Root Operations That Put in/Put Back or Move Some/All of a Body Part
- Root Operations That Alter the Diameter/Route of a Tubular Body Part
- Root Operations That Always Involve a Device
- Root Operations Involving Examination Only
- Root Operations That Define Other Repairs
- Root Operations That Define Other Objectives

Root Operations That Take Out Some or All of a Body Part

Refer to page 489 in the *ICD-10-PCS 2011 Code Book*, Appendix B.

The five root operations belonging to this group are:

- Excision (B)
- Resection (T)
- Detachment (6)
- Destruction (5)
- Extraction (D)

Excision – Root Operation B

Excision B	Definition	Cutting out or off, without replacement, a portion of a body part
	Explanation	The qualifier **Diagnostic** is used to identify excision procedures that are biopsies
	Examples	Partial nephrectomy, liver biopsy, breast lumpectomy, breast reduction for medical reasons (for cosmetic reasons is Alteration), Excisional debridement (non-excisional debridement is Extraction)

Excision is coded when a portion of a body part is cut out or off using a sharp instrument. All root operations that employ cutting to accomplish the objective allow the use of any sharp instrument, including but not limited to:

- Scalpel
- Wire
- Scissors
- Bone saw
- Electrocautery tip

-Extraction

Coding Note: Bone Marrow and Endometrial Biopsies
Bone marrow and endometrial biopsies are not coded to **Excision**. They are coded to **Extraction**, with the qualifier Diagnostic.

Coding Guideline B3.9. Excision for Graft
If an autograft is obtained from a different body part in order to complete the objective of the procedure, a separate procedure is coded.

Example: Coronary bypass with excision of saphenous vein graft, excision of saphenous vein is coded separately

Additional examples of Excision procedures:

- Excision sebaceous cyst right buttock
- Excision malignant melanoma from skin right ear
- Laparoscopy with excision of endometrial implant from left ovary
- EGD with gastric biopsy
- Open endarterectomy of left common carotid artery
- Excision of basal cell carcinoma of lower lip
- Open excision of tail of pancreas
- Percutaneous biopsy of right gastrocnemius muscle
- Open excision of lesion from right Achilles tendon

2.1. Excision of malignant melanoma from the skin of the left upper arm, and right hand

Code(s): 0HBCX22 0HBFX22

2.2. Percutaneous needle core biopsy (diagnostic) of the left kidney pelvis

Code(s): ______________________________

2.3. Sigmoidoscopy with sigmoid polypectomy

Code(s): ______________________________

Resection – Root Operation T

Resection T	Definition	Cutting out or off, without replacement, all of a body part
	Explanation	N/A
	Examples	Total nephrectomy, total lobectomy of lung, total mastectomy

Resection is similar to **Excision** except **Resection** includes all of a body part, or any subdivision of a body part that has its own body part value in ICD-10-PCS, while **Excision** includes only a portion of a body part.

Coding Note: Lymph Nodes
When an entire lymph node chain is cut out, the appropriate root operation is **Resection**. When a lymph node(s) is cut out, the root operation is **Excision**.

Coding Note: Documentation
There is an opportunity to provide physician education on the need for more complete documentation in the medical record on the following:

- Lymph node(s) versus the complete chain
- The complete body part removal versus a portion

Coding Guideline B3.8 Excision versus Resection
PCS contains specific body parts for anatomical subdivisions of a body part, such as lobes of the lungs or liver and regions of the intestine. Resection of the specific body part is coded whenever all of the body part is cut out or off, rather than coding Excision of a less specific body part.

Example: Left upper lung lobectomy is coded to Resection of Upper Lung Lobe, Left rather than Excision of Lung, Left.

Additional examples of Resection procedures:

- Right hemicolectomy
- Open resection of cecum
- Total excision of pituitary gland
- Explantation of left failed kidney
- Open left axillary total lymphadenectomy
- Laparoscopic-assisted total vaginal hysterectomy
- Open resection of papillary muscle
- Radical open retropubic prostatectomy
- Laparoscopic cholecystectomy
- Endoscopic bilateral total maxillary sinusectomy

2.4. Open resection of descending colon

Code(s): ____________________

Coding Guideline B3.4. Biopsy Followed by More Definitive Treatment
If a diagnostic Excision, Extraction, or Drainage procedure (biopsy) is followed by a more definitive procedure, such as Destruction, Excision, or Resection at the same procedure site, both the biopsy and the more definitive treatment are coded.

2.5. Percutaneous needle biopsy of right breast followed by right total mastectomy, open

Code(s): 0HBT3ZX 0HTT0ZZ

2.6. Laparoscopic cholecystectomy converted to complete cholecystectomy, open

Code(s): 0FT40ZZ 0FJ44ZZ

2.7. Open right axillary lymphadenectomy of the complete chain

Code(s): 07T50ZZ

Detachment – Root Operation 6

Detachment 6	Definition	Cutting off all or part of the upper or lower extremities
	Explanation	The body part value is the site of the detachment, with a qualifier, if applicable, to further specify the level where the extremity was detached
	Examples	Below knee amputation, disarticulation of shoulder, amputation above elbow

Detachment represents a narrow range of procedures; it is used exclusively for amputation procedures. **Detachment** procedure codes are found only in body systems X, Anatomical Regions, Upper Extremities and Y, Anatomic Regions, Lower Extremities because amputations are performed on extremities across overlapping body layers and so could not be coded to a specific musculoskeletal body system such as the bones or joints.

Coding Note: Detachment Qualifiers
The specific qualifiers used for **Detachment** are dependent on the body part value in the upper and lower extremities body systems.

Refer to Qualifiers on pages 554–555 of the *ICD-10-PCS 2011 Code Book*, Appendix F: Character Meanings – Anatomical Regions, Upper and Lower Extremities (X and Y).

In addition, the following definitions have been developed for these qualifiers. (These definitions are only available in the ICD-10-PCS Reference Manual.)

Body Part	**Qualifier**	**Definition**
Upper arm and upper leg	1	High: Amputation at the proximal portion of the shaft of the humerus or femur
	2	Mid: Amputation at the middle portion of the shaft of the humerus or femur
	3	Low: Amputation at the distal portion of the shaft of the humerus or femur

Note: The same definitions would be utilized for lower arm and leg.

Coding Note: Documentation
There is an opportunity to provide physician education on the need for more complete documentation in the medical record on the actual location of the amputation. According to the definition the coding professional needs to know if the amputation is at the proximal, middle or distal portion of the *shaft* of the humerus, femur, radius/ulna or tibia/fibula.

Body Part	Qualifier	Definition
Hand and foot	0	Complete
	4	Complete 1st Ray
	5	Complete 2nd Ray
	6	Complete 3rd Ray
	7	Complete 4th Ray
	8	Complete 5th Ray
	9	Partial 1st Ray
	B	Partial 2nd Ray
	C	Partial 3rd Ray
	D	Partial 4th Ray
	F	Partial 5th Ray

When coding amputation of Hand and Foot the following definitions are followed:

- **Complete:** Amputation through the carpometacarpal joint of the hand, or through the tarsal-metatarsal joint of the foot.
- **Partial:** Amputation anywhere along the shaft or head of the metacarpal bone of the hand, or of the metatarsal bone of the foot.

Body Part	Qualifier	Definition
Thumb, finger, or toe	0	Complete: Amputation at the metacarpophalangeal/metatarsal-phalangeal joint
	1	High: Amputation anywhere along the proximal phalanx
	2	Mid: Amputation through the proximal interphalangeal joint or anywhere along the middle phalanx
	3	Low: Amputation through the distal interphalangeal joint or anywhere along the distal phalanx

Coding Note: Qualifier Value

When a surgeon uses the word "toe" to describe the amputation, but the operative report says he extends the amputation to the midshaft of the fifth metatarsal, which is the foot, the qualifier is Partial 5th Ray.

Additional examples of Detachment procedures:

- Fifth toe ray amputation
- Fifth ray carpometacarpal joint amputation of left hand
- Right leg and hip amputation through ischium
- DIP joint amputation of right thumb
- Right wrist joint amputation
- Mid-shaft amputation of right humerus
- Left fourth toe amputation at mid-proximal phalanx
- Right above-knee amputation of distal femur

2.8. Amputation at left elbow level

Code(s): ____

2.9. Right ankle joint amputation

Code(s): 0Y6M0Z0

2.10. Transmetatarsal amputation of foot at right big toe

Code(s): ____________________

Destruction – Root Operation 5

Destruction 5	Definition	Physical eradication of all or a portion of a body part by the direct use of energy, force, or a destructive agent
	Explanation	None of the body part is physically taken out
	Examples	Fulguration of rectal polyp, cautery of skin lesion, fulguration of endometrium

Destruction "takes out" a body part in the sense that it obliterates the body part so it is no longer there. This root operation defines a broad range of common procedures, since it can be used anywhere in the body to treat a variety of conditions, including:

- Skin and genital warts
- Nasal and colon polyps
- Esophageal varices
- Endometrial implants
- Nerve lesions

Coding Note: Usually there would be no pathology report present for Destruction procedures because it is destroyed or obliterated. Occasionally, tissue remains in an instrument, and may be sent to pathology.

Additional examples of Destruction procedures:

- Radiofrequency coagulation of trigeminal nerve
- Percutaneous radiofrequency ablation of right vocal cord lesion
- Cautery of nosebleed
- Cautery of oozing varicose vein of left calf
- Laparoscopy with destruction of endometriosis on both ovaries
- Laser percutaneous coagulation of right retinal vessel hemorrhage
- Talc injection pleurodesis, left side
- Sclerotherapy of brachial plexus lesion with alcohol injection
- Fulguration of endometrium

2.11. Laparoscopy with ablation of endometriosis, endometrium, and bilateral fallopian tubes

Code(s): 0U5BH22 0U57H22

2.12. Left heart catheterization with laser destruction of arrhythmogenic focus, A-V node

Code(s): ______________________________

2.13. Cryotherapy of three warts on left hand and one wart on right hand

Code(s): 0H5GXZD 0H5FXZZ

Extraction – Root Operation D

Extraction D	Definition	Pulling or stripping out or off all or a portion of a body part by the use of force Bone marrow Bx
	Explanation	The qualifier **Diagnostic** is used to identify extraction procedures that are biopsies
	Examples	Dilation and curettage, vein stripping, phacoemulsification without IOL implant (phacoemulsification with IOL implant is Replacement), non-excisional debridement (excisional debridement is excision), liposuction for medical reasons (liposuction for cosmetic reasons is Alteration)

Extraction is coded when the method employed to take out the body part is pulling or stripping. Minor cutting, such as that used in vein stripping procedures, is included in **Extraction** if the objective of the procedure is nevertheless met by pulling or stripping. As with all applicable ICD-10-PCS codes, cutting used to reach the procedure site is specified in the approach value.

Coding Note: Documentation
Be careful of documentation. It is important to convert common terminology to the appropriate root operation according to the intent of the procedure. For example, the procedure documentation may **say** removal, but in actuality, using PCS definitions, an extraction was performed. Removal of a thumbnail would be coded to Extraction. The root operation of Removal is not correct because by definition a Removal in ICD-10-PCS is defined as taking out or off a device from a body part.

Additional examples of Extraction procedures:

- Extraction of teeth
- Suction dilation & curettage
- Removal left thumbnail
- Phacoemulsification cataract without replacement
    - A phacoemulsification with IOL implant is classified to the root operation Replacement. Remember that this group of root operations includes taking out, but not replacement.
- Laparoscopy with needle aspiration of ova for in-vitro fertilization
- Non-excisional debridement of skin ulcer, right foot
    - An excisional debridement is classified to the root operation Excision.
- Open stripping of abdominal fascia, right side
- Hysteroscopy with D&C
- Liposuction for medical purposes, left upper arm
    - A liposuction for cosmetic reasons is coded to the root operation Alteration.
- Removal of tattered right ear drum fragments with tweezers
- Microincisional phlebectomy of spider veins, right lower leg
- Bone marrow biopsy
- Endometrial biopsy (See note in Excision section.)

2.14. Non-excisional debridement of skin ulcer of back

Code(s): ______________________________

2.15. Forceps total mouth extraction, lower and upper teeth

Code(s): ______________________________

2.16. Liposuction for medical purposes, right upper leg

Code(s): 0JDL3ZZ

Root Operations That Take Out Solids, Fluids, or Gases from a Body Part

Refer to page 490 in the *ICD-10-PCS 2011 Code Book*, Appendix B.

The three root operations belonging to this group are:

- Drainage (9)
- Extirpation (C)
- Fragmentation (F)

Drainage – Root Operation 9

Drainage 9	Definition	Taking or letting out fluids and/or gases from a body part
	Explanation	The qualifier **Diagnostic** is used to identify drainage procedures that are biopsies
	Examples	Thoracentesis, Incision and Drainage, Aspiration, Lumbar puncture

The root operation **Drainage** is coded for both diagnostic and therapeutic drainage procedures. When drainage is accomplished by putting in a catheter, the device value **Drainage Device** is coded in the sixth character.

Additional examples of Drainage procedures:

- Routine Foley catheter placement
- Laparoscopy with right ovarian cystotomy and drainage
- Laparotomy with hepatotomy and drain placement for liver abscess, left lobe
- Thoracentesis of left pleural effusion
- Percutaneous chest tube placement for right pneumothorax
- Urinary nephrostomy catheter placement
- Endoscopic drainage of right ethmoid sinus

Coding Guideline B4.1b Body Part General Guidelines
If the prefix "peri" is combined with a body part to identify the site of the procedure, the procedure is coded to the body part named.

Example: A procedure site identified as perirenal is coded to the kidney body part.

2.17. Incision and drainage of external perianal abscess

Code(s): ______________________________

2.18. Open right hip arthrotomy with drain placement

Code(s): 0S9900Z

2.19. Diagnostic percutaneous paracentesis for ascites

Code(s): ______________________________

Extirpation – Root Operation C

Extirpation C	Definition	Taking or cutting out solid matter from a body part.
	Explanation	The solid matter may be an abnormal byproduct of a biological function or a foreign body; it may be imbedded in a body part, or in the lumen of a tubular body part. The solid matter may or may not have been previously broken into pieces.
	Examples	Thrombectomy, endarterectomy, choledocholithotomy, excision foreign body.

Extirpation represents a range of procedures where the body part itself is not the focus of the procedure. Instead, the objective is to remove solid material such as a foreign body, thrombus, or calculus from the body part.

Additional examples of Extirpation procedures:

- Foreign body removal, skin
- De-clotting of arteriovenous dialysis graft
- Removal of foreign body, left cornea
- Esophagogastroscopy with removal of bezoar from stomach
- Transurethral cystoscopy with removal of bladder calculus
- Laparoscopy with excision of old suture from mesentery
- Incision and removal of right lacrimal duct calculus
- Non-incisional removal of intraluminal foreign body from vagina
- Open excision of retained foreign body, subcutaneous tissue of left foot

Coding Guideline B4.2. Branches of Body Parts
Where a specific branch of a body part does not have its own body part value in PCS, the body part is coded to the closest proximal branch that has a specific body part value.

Example: A procedure performed on the mandibular branch of the trigeminal nerve is coded to the trigeminal nerve body part value.

Coding Guideline B4.7. Fingers and Toes
If a body system does not contain a separate body part value for fingers, procedures performed on the fingers are coded to the body part value for the hand. If a body system does not contain a separate body part value for toes, procedures performed on the toes are coded to the body part value for the foot

Example: Excision of finger muscle is coded to one of the hand muscle body part values in the Muscles body system.

2.20. Percutaneous mechanical thrombectomy, right common interosseous artery

Code(s): 03C9322

2.21. Forceps removal of foreign body in the left nostril

Code(s): 09CKX22 ____________________

2.22. Foreign body removal, skin of right index finger

Code(s): ____________________

Fragmentation – Root Operation F

Fragmentation F	Definition	Breaking solid matter in a body part into pieces.
	Explanation	The physical force (for example, manual, ultrasonic) applied directly or indirectly is used to break the solid matter into pieces. The solid matter may be an abnormal byproduct of a biological function or a foreign body. The pieces of solid matter are not taken out.
	Examples	Extracorporeal shockwave lithotripsy, transurethral lithotripsy.

Fragmentation is coded for procedures to break up, but not remove, solid material such as a calculus or foreign body. This root operation includes both direct and extracorporeal **Fragmentation** procedures.

Additional examples of Fragmentation procedures:

- Hysteroscopy with intraluminal lithotripsy of left fallopian tube calcification
- Thoracotomy with crushing of pericardial calcifications
- Extracorporeal shockwave lithotripsy (ESWL) of left kidney

Coding Guideline B4.3. Bilateral Body Part Values
Bilateral body part values are available for a limited number of body parts. If the identical procedure is performed on contralateral body parts, and a bilateral body part value exists for that body part, a single procedure is coded using the bilateral body part value. If no bilateral body part value exists, code each procedure separately using the appropriate body part value.

Coding Guideline B3.11a. Inspection Procedures
Inspection of a body part(s) performed in order to achieve the objective of a procedure is not coded separately.

2.23. ESWL, bilateral ureters

Code(s): ____________________

2.24. Transurethral cystoscopy with fragmentation of bladder neck calculus

Code(s): 0TFC822

2.25. ERCP with lithotripsy of common bile duct stone

Code(s): 0FF9822

Root Operations Involving Cutting or Separation Only

Refer to page 491 in the *ICD-10-PCS 2011 Code Book*, Appendix B.

The two root operations belonging to this group are:

- Division (8)
- Release (N)

Division – Root Operation 8

Division 8	Definition	Cutting into a body part without draining fluids and/or gases from the body part in order to separate or transect a body part
	Explanation	All or a portion of the body part is separated into two or more portions
	Examples	Spinal cordotomy, osteotomy, neurotomy, episiotomy

The root operation **Division** is coded when the objective of the procedure is to cut into, transect, or otherwise separate all or a portion of a body part. When the objective is to cut or separate the area around a body part, the attachments to a body part, or between subdivisions of a body part that are causing abnormal constraint, the root operation **Release** is coded instead.

Coding Guideline B3.14. Release vs. Division
If the sole objective of the procedure is freeing a body part without cutting the body part, the root operation is Release. If the sole objective of the procedure is separating or transecting a body part, the root operation is Division.

Examples: Freeing a nerve root from surrounding scar tissue to relieve pain is coded to the root operation Release. Severing a nerve root to relieve pain is coded to the root operation Division.

Additional examples of Division procedures:

- Left heart catheterization with division of bundle of HIS
- Sacral rhizotomy for pain control, percutaneous
- Anal sphincterotomy
- EGD with esophagotomy of esophagogastric junction

Coding Guideline B4.1a. Body Part Guideline
If a procedure is performed on a portion of a body part that does not have a separate body part value, code the body part value corresponding to the whole body part.

Coding Guideline B3.2.b. Multiple Procedures During the same operative episode, multiple procedures are coded if the same root operation is repeated at different body sites that are included in the same body part value. *Example*: Excision of the sartorius muscle and excision of the gracilis muscle are both included in the Upper Leg Muscle body part value, and multiple procedures are coded.

2.26. Open osteotomy of the capitate and lunate bones, right hand

Code(s): ____________________

Coding Guideline B4.5. Tendons, Ligaments, Bursae and Fascia near a Joint Procedures performed on tendons, ligaments, bursae and fascia supporting a joint are coded to the body part in the respective body system that is the focus of the procedure. Procedures performed on joint structures themselves are coded to the body part in the joint body systems. *Example:* Repair of the anterior cruciate ligament of the knee is coded to the knee bursae and ligament body part in the bursae and ligaments body system. Knee arthroscopy with shaving of articular cartilage is coded to the Knee Joint body part in the Lower Joints body system.

2.27. Division of left Achilles tendon, percutaneous

Code(s): ____________________

Release – Root Operation N

Release N	Definition	Freeing a body part from an abnormal physical constraint by cutting or by use of force
	Explanation	Some of the restraining tissue may be taken out but none of the body part is taken out
	Examples	Adhesiolysis, carpal tunnel release, manipulation of joint adhesions

The objective of procedures represented in the root operation **Release** is to free a body part from abnormal constraint. **Release** procedures are coded to the body part being freed. The procedure can be performed on the area around a body part, on the attachments to a body part, or between subdivisions of a body part that are causing the abnormal constraint.

Coding Guideline B3.13. Release Procedures
In the root operation Release, the body part value coded is the body part being freed and not the tissue being manipulated or cut to free the body part.

Example: Lysis of intestinal adhesions is coded to the specific intestine body part value.

Additional examples of Release procedures:

- Incision of scar contracture, left elbow
- Open posterior tarsal tunnel release
- Manual rupture of left shoulder joint adhesions under general anesthesia
- Laparoscopy with lysis of peritoneal adhesions
- Mitral valvulotomy for release of fused leaflets, open
- Frenulotomy for treatment of tongue-tie syndrome

2.28. Right shoulder arthroscopy with coracoacromial ligament release

Code(s): ______________________________

2.29. Laparoscopy with freeing of bilateral ovaries and fallopian tubes

Code(s): ______________________________

2.30. Right open carpal tunnel release

Code(s): 01N50ZZ

Root Operations That Put In/Put Back or Move Some/ All of a Body Part

Refer to page 489 in the *ICD-10-PCS 2011 Code Book*, Appendix B.

The four root operations belonging to this group are:

- Transplantation (Y)
- Reattachment (M)
- Transfer (X)
- Reposition (S)

Transplantation – Root Operation Y

Transplantation Y	Definition	Putting in or on all or a portion of a living body part taken from another individual or animal to physically take the place and/or function of all or a portion of a similar body part
	Explanation	The native body part may or may not be taken out, and the transplanted body part may take over all or a portion of its function
	Examples	Kidney transplant, heart transplant

A small number of procedures is represented in the root operation **Transplantation** and includes only the body parts currently being transplanted. Qualifier values specify the genetic compatibility of the body part transplanted.

Coding Guideline B3.16. Transplantation vs. Administration
Putting in a mature and functioning living body part taken from another individual or animal is coded to the root operation Transplantation. Putting in autologous or nonautologous cells is coded to the Administration section.

Example: Putting in autologous or nonautologous bone marrow, pancreatic islet cells, or stem cells is coded to the Administration section.

Coding Note: Bone Marrow Transplant
Bone marrow transplant procedures are coded in section 3, Administration, to the root operation 2, Transfusion

In the Tables for Transplant Procedures, the Qualifier values are:

- Allogeneic
- Syngeneic
- Zooplastic

The following table provides definitions of these terms.

Qualifier Choices Character 7

Type of Transplant	Qualifier Character	Definition
Allogeneic	0	Taken from different individuals of the same species
Syngeneic	1	Having to do with individuals or tissues that have identical genes, such as identical twins
Zooplastic	2	Tissue from an animal to a human

Additional examples of Transplantation procedures:

- Open transplant of large intestine, organ donor match
- Left kidney and pancreas transplant, open, organ bank transplant
- Orthotopic heart transplant using porcine heart, open

2.31. Liver transplant with donor matched liver

Code(s): 0FY00Z0

2.32. Bilateral lung transplant, open, using an organ donor match

Code(s): 0BYM0Z0

Reattachment – Root Operation M

Reattachment M	Definition	Putting back in or on all or a portion of a separated body part to its normal location or other suitable location
	Explanation	Vascular circulation and nervous pathways may or may not be reestablished
	Examples	Reattachment of hand, reattachment of avulsed kidney, reattachment of finger

Procedures coded to **Reattachment** include putting back a body part that has been cut off or avulsed. Nerves and blood vessels may or may not be reconnected in a **Reattachment** procedure.

Additional examples of Reattachment procedures:

- Complex reattachment of left index finger
- Replantation of avulsed scalp
- Reattachment of traumatic right gastrocnemius avulsion, open
- Closed replantation of three avulsed teeth, upper jaw

2.33. Reattachment of severed left ear

Code(s): 09M1XZZ

2.34. Reattachment of severed right hand

Code(s): 0XMJ0ZZ

Transfer – Root Operation X

Transfer X Pivot must stay connected	Definition	Moving, without taking out, all or a portion of a body part to another location to take over the function of all or a portion of a body part
	Explanation	The body part transferred remains connected to its vascular and nervous supply
	Examples	Tendon transfer, skin pedicle flap transfer, skin transfer flap

Coding Note: Free grafts are coded to the root operation of Replacement.

The root operation **Transfer** is used to represent procedures where a body part is moved to another location without disrupting its vascular and nervous supply. In the body systems that classify the subcutaneous tissue, fascia, and muscle body parts, a qualifier is used to specify when more than one tissue layer was used in the transfer procedure, such as musculocutaneous flap transfer.

Coding Note: Body System Value
The body system value describes the deepest tissue layer in the flap. The qualifier can be used to describe the other tissue layers, if any, being transferred.

Additional examples of Transfer procedures:

- Right scalp advancement flap to right temple
- Transfer right index finger to right thumb position, open
- Fasciocutaneous flap closure of left upper arm, open
- Trigeminal to fascial nerve transfer, percutaneous endoscopic
- Left leg flexor digitorum longus tendon transfer, percutaneous endoscopic
- Right wrist palmaris longus tendon transfer, open

2.35. Left foot open flexor digitorum brevis tendon transfer

Code(s): 0LXW0ZZ

2.36. Endoscopic radial to median nerve transfer

Code(s): __________

2.37. Skin transfer flap closure of complex open wound, left chest

Code(s): 0HX5XZZ

Reposition – Root Operation S

Reposition S	Definition	Moving to its normal location or other suitable location all or a portion of a body part.
	Explanation	The body part is moved to a new location from an abnormal location, or from a normal location where it is not functioning correctly. The body part may or may not be cut out or off to be moved to the new location.
	Examples	Reposition of undescended testicle, fracture reduction.

Reposition represents procedures for moving a body part to a new location. The range of **Reposition** procedures includes moving a body part to its normal location, or moving a body part to a new location to enhance its ability to function.

> **Coding Guideline B3.15. Reposition for Fracture Treatment**
> Reduction of a displaced fracture is coded to the root operation Reposition and the application of a cast or splint in conjunction with the Reposition procedure is not coded separately. Treatment of a nondisplaced fracture is coded to the procedure performed.
>
> *Examples:* 1. Putting a pin in a nondisplaced fracture is coded to the root operation Insertion.
> 2. Casting of a nondisplaced fracture is coded to the root operation Immobilization in the Placement section.

> **Coding Note:** The diagnosis code in ICD-10-CM would reflect that a displaced fracture is being reduced when the root operation of Reposition is used.

Additional examples of Reposition procedures:

- Open fracture reduction with internal fixation, left tibia and ulna
- Open fracture reduction, displaced fracture of right distal humerus
- Closed reduction with percutaneous internal fixation of left femoral neck fracture
- Right knee arthroscopy with reposition of patellar ligament
- Open transposition of ulnar nerve
- Laparoscopy with gastropexy for malrotation

2.38. Relocation of bilateral undescended testicle, percutaneous

Code(s): ______________________________

2.39. Open fracture reduction, displaced fracture of right humeral head

Code(s): ______________________________

2.40. Right knee arthroscopy with reposition of anterior cruciate ligament

Code(s): ~~0SSC4ZZ~~ 0MSN4ZZ

2.41. Closed reduction with percutaneous internal fixation of displaced left intertrochanteric femoral fracture

Code(s): ______________________________

Root Operations That Alter the Diameter/Route of a Tubular Body Part

Refer to page 490 in the *ICD-10-PCS 2011 Code Book*, Appendix B.

The four root operations belonging to this group are:

- Restriction (V)
- Occlusion (L)
- Dilation (7)
- Bypass (1)

Restriction – Root Operation V

Restriction V	Definition	Partially closing an orifice or the lumen of a tubular body part
	Explanation	The orifice can be a natural orifice or an artificially-created orifice
	Examples	Esophagogastric fundoplication, cervical cerclage

The root operation **Restriction** is coded when the objective of the procedure is to narrow the diameter of a tubular body part or orifice. **Restriction** includes either intraluminal or extraluminal methods for narrowing the diameter.

Additional examples of Restriction Procedures:

- Thoracotomy with banding of left pulmonary artery with extraluminal device
- Restriction of thoracic duct with intraluminal stent
- Non-incisional, trans-nasal placement of restrictive stent in lacrimal duct

Coding Note: Since intraluminal or extraluminal clips are frequently used to accomplish the objectives of Restriction and Occlusion procedures, careful review of the operative report is required. Research on the procedure technique may also be helpful.

2.42. Transvaginal cervical cerclage using McDonald technique

Code(s): ______________________________

2.43. Clipping of anterior cerebral artery aneurysm via craniotomy

Code(s): 03VG0CZ

Occlusion – Root Operation L

Occlusion L	Definition	Completely closing an orifice or the lumen of a tubular body part
	Explanation	The orifice can be a natural orifice or an artificially created orifice
	Examples	Fallopian tube ligation, ligation of inferior vena cava

The root operation **Occlusion** is coded when the objective of the procedure is to close off a tubular body part or orifice. **Occlusion** includes both intraluminal and extraluminal methods of closing off the body part. Division of the tubular body part prior to closing it is an integral part of the **Occlusion** procedure.

Coding Guideline B3.12. Occlusion vs. Restriction for Vessel Embolization Procedures
If the objective of an embolization procedure is to completely close a vessel, the root operation Occlusion is coded. If the objective of an embolization procedure is to narrow the lumen of a vessel, the root operation Restriction is coded.

Examples: 1. Tumor embolization is coded to the root operation Occlusion, because the objective of the procedure is to cut off the blood supply to the vessel.
2. Embolization of a cerebral aneurysm is coded to the root operation Restriction, because the objective of the procedure is not to close off the vessel entirely, but to narrow the lumen of the vessel at the site of the aneurysm where it is abnormally wide.

Research on embolizations may be required to gain additional information about how the procedure is performed. The purpose of an embolization is to prevent blood flow to an area of the body. It is used during hemorrhage (i.e., arteriovenous [AV] malformation, cerebral aneurysms, GI bleeding, epistaxis, post-partum hemorrhage). However, the procedure has other uses, such as in the treatment of tumors and disorders of the portal vein. An artificial embolus is introduced (coils, particles, foam, plugs). Some of the common agents used to do this are sclerosing agents, ethanol, or Gelfoam. In order to code occlusions and restrictions correctly, the coder must know if it is complete or partial, and physician documentation or additional physician query is essential.

Additional examples of Occlusion procedures:

- Uterine artery embolization(completely closing the vessel)
- Ligation of esophageal vein
- Complete embolization of internal carotid-cavernous fistula
- Complete embolization of vascular supply of intracranial meningioma

2.44. Laparoscopy with bilateral occlusion of fallopian tubes using extraluminal clips

Code(s): 0UL74CZ

2.45. Percutaneous ligation of left external jugular vein

Code(s): ____

2.46. Open suture ligation of failed AV graft, right brachial artery

Code(s): ____

Dilation – Root Operation 7

Dilation 7	Definition	Expanding an orifice or the lumen of a tubular body part.
	Explanation	The orifice can be a natural orifice or an artificially created orifice. Accomplished by stretching a tubular body part using intraluminal pressure or by cutting part of the orifice or wall of the tubular body part.
	Examples	Percutaneous transluminal angioplasty, percutaneous transluminal coronary angioplasty (PTCA), laryngeal stenosis dilation, dilation common bile duct.

The root operation **Dilation** is coded when the objective of the procedure is to enlarge the diameter of a tubular body part or orifice. **Dilation** includes both intraluminal and extraluminal methods of enlarging the diameter. A device placed to maintain the new diameter is an integral part of the **Dilation** procedure, and is coded to a sixth-character device value in the **Dilation** procedure code.

Coding Guideline B4.4. Coronary Arteries
The coronary arteries are classified as a single body part that is further specified by number of sites treated and not by name or number of arteries. Separate body part values are used to specify the number of sites treated when the same procedure is performed on multiple sites in the coronary arteries.

Examples: 1. Angioplasty of two distinct sites in the left anterior descending coronary artery with placement of two stents is coded as Dilation of Coronary Arteries, Two Sites, with Intraluminal Device. 2. Angioplasty of two distinct sites in the left anterior descending coronary artery, one with stent placed and one without, is coded separately as Dilation of Coronary Artery, One Site with Intraluminal Device, and Dilation of Coronary Artery, One Site with No Device.

Coding Note: In ICD-10-PCS, the classification of the coronary arteries is as a single body part. It doesn't matter what the number of arteries treated is (that is, right coronary artery, left anterior descending, or left circumflex, or the branches). The distinguishing factor is the **number of sites treated**.

During PTAs and PTCAs the narrowed or obstructed blood vessel is mechanically widened. Typically, a collapsed balloon on a guide wire (balloon catheter) is passed into the narrowed locations and then inflated. The balloon crushes the fatty deposits, and then the balloon is collapsed and withdrawn. When a device is placed, it is identified by the sixth-character. The device values are:

- Drug-eluting intraluminal device
- Intraluminal device
- Radioactive intraluminal device

Additional examples of Dilation procedures:

- Cystoscopy with intraluminal dilation of bladder neck stricture
- Dilation of old anastomosis of femoral artery
- Dilation upper esophageal stricture using Bougie sound
- PTA brachial artery stenosis
- Trans-nasal dilation and stent placement lacrimal duct
- Hysteroscopy with balloon dilation of fallopian tubes
- Tracheoscopy with intraluminal dilation of tracheal stenosis
- Cystoscopy with dilation of ureteral stricture, with stent placement

2.47. ERCP with balloon dilation of common bile duct

Code(s): ____________________

2.48. PTA of right radial artery stenosis

Code(s): 037B3ZZ

2.49. Laryngoscopy with intraluminal dilation of laryngeal stenosis

Code(s): ____________________

2.50. PTCA of two coronary arteries. RCA with stent and LAD without stent

Code(s): 02703DZ 02703ZZ

Bypass – Root Operation 1

Bypass 1	Definition	Altering the route of passage of the contents of a tubular body part
	Explanation	Rerouting content of a body part to a downstream area of the normal route, to a similar route and body part, or to an abnormal route and dissimilar body part. Includes one or more anastomoses, with or without the use of a device
	Examples	Coronary artery bypass graft (CABG), colostomy formation

Bypass is coded when the objective of the procedure is to reroute the contents of a tubular body part. The range of **Bypass** procedures includes normal routes such as those made in coronary artery bypass procedures, and abnormal routes such as those made in colostomy formation procedures.

Coding Guideline B3.6a. Bypass Procedures
Bypass procedures are coded by identifying the body part bypassed "from" and the body part bypassed "to." The fourth character body part specifies the body part bypassed from, and the qualifier specifies the body part bypassed to.

Example: Bypass from stomach to jejunum, stomach is the body part and jejunum is the qualifier.

Coding Guideline B3.6b. Bypass Procedures
Coronary arteries are classified by number of distinct sites treated, rather than number of coronary arteries or anatomic name of a coronary artery (for example, left anterior descending). Coronary artery bypass procedures are coded differently than other bypass procedures as described in the previous guideline. Rather than identifying the body part bypassed from, the body part identifies the number of coronary artery sites bypassed to, and the qualifier specifies the vessel bypassed from.

Example: Aortocoronary artery bypass of one site on the left anterior descending coronary artery and one site on the obtuse marginal coronary artery is classified in the body part axis of classification as two coronary artery sites and the qualifier specifies the aorta as the body part bypassed from.

Coding Guideline B3.6c. Bypass Procedures
If multiple coronary artery sites are bypassed, a separate procedure is coded for each coronary artery site that uses a different device and/or qualifier.

Example: Aortocoronary artery bypass and internal mammary coronary artery bypass are coded separately.

Coding Guideline B3.9. Excision for Graft
If an autograft is obtained from a different body part in order to complete the objective of the procedure, a separate procedure is coded.

Example: Coronary bypass with excision of saphenous vein graft, excision of saphenous vein is coded separately.

Coding Note: Autograft
An autograft is tissue or organ transferred into a new position in the body of the same individual. Synonyms are: autotransplant, autogeneic graft, autologous graft, autoplastic graft (*Stedman's* 2006).

The choices for ~~qualifiers~~ device are autologous, synthetic substitute, or nonautologous tissue substitute. The definitions for each are listed here:

Type of Tissue	~~Qualifier~~ Device Character	Definition
Autologous (vein or artery)	9 or A	Referring to a graft in which the donor and recipient areas are in the same individual
Synthetic Substitute	J	Any type of synthetic substitute
Nonautologous Tissue Substitute	K	Nonautologous allogeneic donor tissue implanted from one human to another

Additional examples of Bypass procedures:

- Aorto-bifemoral bypass
- Temporal artery to intracranial artery bypass using Gore-Tex graft
- Tracheostomy formation with tracheostomy tube placement
- Percutaneous in-situ coronary venous arterialization (PICVA) of single coronary artery
- Femoral-popliteal artery bypass
- Shunting of intrathecal cerebrospinal fluid to peritoneal cavity using synthetic shunt
- Pleuroperitoneal shunt, pleural cavity, using synthetic device

Coding Note: When assigning the device value, the key to remember is that to be considered a device, this needs to be material used as a graft (separated) and not moved over. For example, when the internal mammary is loosened from one side and brought around to the occluded coronary artery, the artery is not used as free graft material—this would be considered no device.

2.51. Open gastric bypass with Roux-en-Y limb to jejunum

Code(s): ______________________________

2.52. Open right femoral-posterior tibial artery bypass using cadaver vein graft

Code(s): ______________________________

2.53. Open urinary diversion, left ureter, using ileal conduit to skin; laser destruction of left ureteral lesion

Code(s): ______________________________

2.54. CABG of LAD using left internal mammary artery, open; off pump

Code(s): ______________________________

2.55. Open coronary artery bypass graft of three coronary arteries using left autologous greater saphenous vein, harvested endoscopically

Code(s): ______________________________

2.56. Colostomy formation, open, descending colon to abdominal wall

Code(s): ______________________________

Root Operations That Always Involve a Device

Refer to page 491 in the *ICD-10-PCS 2011 Code Book*, Appendix B.

The six root operations belonging to this group are:

- Insertion (H)
- Replacement (R)
- Supplement (U)
- Change (2)
- Removal (P)
- Revision (W)

Always has Device

Insertion – Root Operation H

Insertion H	Definition	Putting in a non-biological appliance that monitors, assists, performs, or prevents a physiological function but does not physically take the place of a body part
	Explanation	N/A
	Examples	Insertion of radioactive implant, insertion of central venous catheter

The root operation **Insertion** represents those procedures where the sole objective is to put in a device without doing anything else to a body part. Procedures typical of those coded to **Insertion** include putting in a vascular catheter, a pacemaker lead, or a tissue expander.

Additional examples of Insertion procedures:

- Port-A-Cath placement
- Open placement of dual chamber pacemaker in chest wall
- Cystoscopy with placement of brachytherapy seeds in prostate gland
- Percutaneous placement of intrathecal infusion pump for pain management
- Percutaneous placement of Swan-Ganz catheter in superior vena cava
- Open insertion of multiple channel cochlear implant, right ear

2.57. Open placement of single chamber rate responsive pacemaker into the SKIN + subcutaneous tissue of the chest wall

Code(s): 0JH60P1

2.58. Percutaneous insertion of bone growth stimulator electrode, left femoral shaft

Code(s): ______________________

Coding Note: Several electrical bone growth stimulators are available.

- The noninvasive type of stimulator is comprised of coils or electrodes, which are placed on the skin near the fracture site.
- The invasive type includes percutaneous and implanted devices. The percutaneous type involves electrode wires inserted through the skin into the bone while implanted devices include a generator placed under the skin or in the muscles near the gap between the ends of the bones, which have not fused. The implanted devices are surgically placed and later surgically removed.

2.59. Percutaneous placement of pacemaker lead into left atrium

Code(s): ____

Replacement – Root Operation R

Replacement R		
	Definition	Putting in or on biological or synthetic material that physically takes the place and/or function of all or a portion of a body part.
	Explanation	The body part may have been taken out or replaced, or may be taken out, physically eradicated, or rendered nonfunctional during the **Replacement** procedure. **A Removal procedure is coded for taking out the device used in a previous replacement procedure.**
	Examples	Total hip replacement, bone graft, free skin graft, phacoemulsification with IOL implant (phaco without IOL implant is extraction), heart valve replacement, replacement cornea, free TRAM.

The objective of procedures coded to the root operation **Replacement** is to put in a device that takes the place of some or all of a body part. **Replacement** encompasses a wide range of procedures, from joint replacements to grafts of all kinds.

Coding Note: Replacement includes taking out the body part.

Additional examples of Replacement procedures:

- Phacoemulsification of cataract of right eye with intraocular lens implantation
- Right hip hemiarthroplasty, open
- Excision of abdominal aorta with Gore-Tex graft replacement, open
- Open tenonectomy with graft to left ankle using cadaver graft
- Right total hip replacement, open
- Partial-thickness skin graft to right lower leg, autograft

2.60. Total left knee arthroplasty with insertion of total knee prosthesis

Code(s): ______________________________

2.61. Penetrating keratoplasty of left cornea with donor matched cornea, percutaneous approach

Code(s): ______________________________

2.62. Right mastectomy with free TRAM flap reconstruction

Code(s): 0HRT076

2.63. Aortic valve replacement using porcine valve, open

Code(s): 02RF08Z

Supplement – Root Operation U

Supplement U	Definition	Putting in or on biologic or synthetic material that physically reinforces and/or augments the function of a portion of a body part.
	Explanation	The biological material is non-living, or is living and from the same individual. The body part may have been previously replaced, and the **Supplement** procedure is performed to physically reinforce and/or augment the function of the replaced body part.
	Examples	Herniorrhaphy using mesh (herniorrhaphy without mesh is Repair), free nerve graft, mitral valve ring annuloplasty, put a new acetabular liner in a previous hip replacement, abdominal wall herniorrhaphy using mesh.

The objective of procedures coded to the root operation **Supplement** is to put in a device that reinforces or augments the functions of some or all of a body part. The body part may have been taken out during a previous procedure, but is not taken out as part of the **Supplement** procedure. **Supplement** includes a wide range of procedures, from hernia repairs using mesh reinforcement to heart valve annuloplasties and grafts such as nerve grafts that supplement but do not physically take the place of the existing body part.

Additional examples of Supplement procedures:

- Open mitral valve annuloplasty using ring
- Percutaneous endoscopic autograft nerve graft to left radial nerve
- Implantation of CorCap cardiac support device, open
- Open abdominal wall hernia repair using synthetic mesh
- Open tendon graft using autograft
- Onlay lamellar keratoplasty of right cornea using autograft, external approach
- Open resurfacing procedure on left acetabular surface

2.64. Laparoscopic right inguinal hernia repair with Marlex mesh

Code(s): ______________________

2.65. Open anterior colporrhaphy with polypropylene mesh reinforcement

Code(s): ______________________

2.66. Open exchange of liner in right femoral component on previous hip replacement

Code(s): ______________________

Change – Root Operation 2

Change 2	Definition	Taking out or off a device from a body part and putting back an identical or similar device in or on the same body part without cutting or puncturing the skin or a mucous membrane
	Explanation	All **Change** procedures are coded using the approach External
	Examples	Urinary catheter change, gastrostomy tube change, drainage tube change

The root operation **Change** represents only those procedures where a similar device is exchanged without making a new incision or puncture. Typical **Change** procedures include exchange of drainage devices and feeding devices.

Coding Note: Change
In the root operation Change, general body part values are used when the *specific* body part value is not in the table.

Additional examples of Change procedures:

- Percutaneous endoscopic gastrostomy (PEG) tube exchange
- Exchange of cerebral ventriculostomy drainage tube
- Exchange of drainage tube from left hip joint

2.67. Tracheostomy tube exchange

Code(s): 0B21XFZ

2.68. Change chest tube, right pleural cavity (for right pneumothorax)

Code(s): ____________________

2.69. Change Foley urinary catheter

Code(s): ____________________

Removal – Root Operation P

Removal P	Definition	Taking out or off a device from a body part.
	Explanation	If the device is taken out and a similar device is put in without cutting or puncturing the skin or mucous membrane, the procedure is coded to the root operation Change. Otherwise, the procedure for taking out the device is coded to the root operation **Removal**.
	Examples	Drainage tube removal, cardiac pacemaker removal, central line removal.

Removal represents a much broader range of procedures than those for removing the devices contained in the root operation **Insertion**. A procedure to remove a device is coded to **Removal** if it is not an integral part of another root operation and regardless of the approach or the original root operation by which the device was put in.

Coding Note: Removal
In the root operation Removal, general body part values are used when the specific body part value is not in the table.

Additional examples of Removal procedures:

- Removal of tracheostomy tube
- Open removal of lumbar sympathetic neurostimulator
- Non-incisional removal of Swan-Ganz from superior vena cava
- Transurethral removal of brachytherapy seeds
- Incision with removal of K-wire fixation, left second metacarpal

2.70. Removal of endotracheal tube

Code(s): ____________________

2.71. Removal of external fixator, left humeral head fracture

Code(s): ____________________

2.72. Removal of PEG tube (non-incisional)

Code(s): ____________________

2.73. Cystoscopy with retrieval of right ureteral stent

Code(s): ____________________

Revision – Root Operation W

Revision W	Definition	Correcting, to the extent possible, a malfunctioning or displaced device
	Explanation	Revision can include correcting a malfunctioning device by taking out and/or putting in part of the device
	Examples	Adjustment of pacemaker lead, adjustment of hip prosthesis, revision of pacemaker insertion

Revision is coded when the objective of the procedure is to correct the positioning or function of a previously placed device, without taking the entire device out and putting a whole new device in its place. A complete re-do of the original root operation is coded to the root operation that is performed.

Coding Note: Revision
In the root operation Revision, general body part values are used when the specific body part value is not in the table.

Additional examples of Revision procedures:

- Reposition of Swan-Ganz catheter in superior vena cava
- Taking out loose screw and putting larger screw in fracture repair plate, right fibula
- Revision of VAD reservoir placement in chest wall, open

2.74. Open revision of left hip replacement, with readjustment of the prosthesis

Code(s): ____________________

2.75. Adjustment of position, pacemaker lead in left atrium, percutaneous

Code(s): ____________________

Root Operations Involving Examination Only

Refer to page 490 in the *ICD-10-PCS 2011 Code Book*, Appendix B.

The two root operations belonging to this group are:

- Inspection (J)
- Map (K)

Inspection – Root Operation J

Inspection J	Definition	Visually and/or manually exploring a body part
	Explanation	Visual exploration may be performed with or without optical instrumentation. Manual exploration may be performed directly or through intervening body layers
	Examples	Diagnostic arthroscopy, exploratory laparotomy, diagnostic cystoscopy

The root operation **Inspection** represents procedures where the sole objective is to examine a body part. Procedures that are discontinued without any other root operation being performed are also coded to **Inspection**.

Coding Guideline B3.11a. Inspection Procedures
Inspection of a body part(s) performed in order to achieve the objective of a procedure is not coded separately.

Example: Fiberoptic bronchoscopy performed for irrigation of bronchus, only the irrigation procedure is coded.

Coding Guideline B3.11b. Inspection Procedures
If multiple tubular body parts are inspected, the most distal body part inspected is coded. If multiple non-tubular body parts in a region are inspected, the body part that specifies the entire area inspected is coded.

Examples: 1. Cystourethroscopy with inspection of bladder and ureters is coded to the ureter body part value. 2. Exploratory laparotomy with general inspection of abdominal contents is coded to the peritoneal cavity body part value.

Coding Guideline B3.11c. Inspection Procedures
When both an Inspection procedure and another procedure are performed on the same body part during the same episode, if the Inspection procedure is performed using a different approach than the other procedure, the Inspection procedure is coded separately.

Example: Endoscopic inspection of the duodenum is coded separately when open Excision of the duodenum is performed during the same procedural episode.

Coding Note: Procedures that are discontinued without any other root operation being performed are coded to Inspection.

Additional examples of Inspection procedures:

- Diagnostic colposcopy with examination of cervix
- Thoracotomy with exploration of right pleural cavity
- Diagnostic laryngoscopy
- Exploratory arthrotomy left knee
- Colposcopy with diagnostic hysteroscopy
- Endoscopy maxillary sinus
- Transurethral diagnostic cystoscopy

2.76. Diagnostic bronchoscopy of the left bronchus

Code(s): 0BJ08ZZ

2.77. Digital rectal exam

Code(s): ______

2.78. Laparotomy with palpation of left lobe of liver

Code(s): 0FJ00ZZ

2.79. Colonoscopy to the descending colon

Code(s): 0DJD8ZZ

2.80. Ureteroscopy with unsuccessful removal of left ureteral stone

Code(s): 0TJ98ZZ

Map – Root Operation K

Map K	Definition	Locating the route of passage of electrical impulses and/or locating functional areas in a body part
	Explanation	Applicable only to the cardiac conduction mechanism and the central nervous system
	Examples	Cardiac mapping, cortical mapping, cardiac electrophysiological study

The root operation of **Map** represents a very narrow range of procedures. Procedures include only cardiac mapping and cortical mapping.

Coding Note: The only two body systems under Map Procedures are the Central Nervous System (00K) and Heart and Great Vessels (02K).

Additional examples of Map procedures:

- Percutaneous mapping of basal ganglia
- Mapping left cerebral hemisphere
- Intraoperative cardiac mapping during open heart surgery

2.81. Heart catheterization with cardiac mapping

Code(s): 02K83ZZ

2.82. Intraoperative whole brain mapping via craniotomy

Code(s): 00K00ZZ

Root Operations That Define Other Repairs

Refer to page 491 in the *ICD-10-PCS 2011 Code Book*, Appendix B.

The two root operations belonging to this group are:

- Control (3)
- Repair (Q)

Control – Root Operation 3

Control 3	Definition	Stopping, or attempting to stop, postprocedural bleeding
	Explanation	The site of the bleeding is coded as an anatomical region and not to a specific body part
	Examples	Control of post-prostatectomy hemorrhage, control of post-tonsillectomy hemorrhage

Control is used to represent a small range of procedures performed to treat postprocedural bleeding. If the following procedures are required to stop the bleeding, then **Control** is not coded separately.

- Bypass
- Detachment
- Excision
- Extraction
- Reposition
- Replacement
- Resection

Coding Guideline B3.7. Control vs. More Definitive Root Operations
The root operation Control is defined as, "Stopping, or attempting to stop, postprocedural bleeding." If an attempt to stop postprocedural bleeding is initially unsuccessful, and to stop the bleeding requires performing any of the definitive root operations Bypass, Detachment, Excision, Extraction, Reposition, Replacement, or Resection, then that root operation is coded instead of Control.

Example: Resection of spleen to stop postprocedural bleeding is coded to Resection instead of Control.

Coding Note: **Control**
Control includes irrigation or evacuation of hematoma done at the operative site. Both irrigation and evacuation may be necessary to clear the operative field and effectively stop the bleeding.

Additional examples of Control procedures:

- Reopening laparotomy site with ligation of arterial bleeder
- Hysteroscopy with cautery of post-hysterectomy oozing and evacuation of clot (This is Control and not Destruction because the intent is to stop postoperative bleeding.)
- Reopening thoracotomy site with drainage and control of post-op hemopericardium
- Arthroscopy with drainage of hemarthrosis at previous operative site of knee

2.83. Open exploration and ligation of post-op arterial bleeder, right upper arm

Code(s): ______________________

2.84. Control of postoperative retroperitoneal bleeding via laparotomy

Code(s): ______________________

Repair – Root Operation Q

Repair Q	Definition	Restoring, to the extent possible, a body part to its normal anatomic structure and function
	Explanation	Used only when the method to accomplish the repair is not one of the other root operations
	Examples	Herniorrhaphy, suture of laceration

The root operation **Repair** represents a broad range of procedures for restoring the anatomic structure of a body part such as suture of lacerations. Repair also functions as the "not elsewhere classified (NEC)" root operation, to be used when the procedure performed does not meet the definition of one of the other root operations. Fixation devices are included for procedures to repair the bones and joints.

Coding Note: Limited NEC Code Options

- ICD-9-CM often designates codes as "not elsewhere classified" or "other specified" versions of a procedure throughout the code set. NEC options are also provided in ICD-10-PCS, but only for specific, limited use.
- In the Medical and Surgical section, two significant NEC options are the root operations value Q, Repair and the device value Y, Other Device.
- The root operation Repair is a true NEC value. It is used only when the procedure performed is not one of the other root operations in the Medical and Surgical section.

Additional examples of Repair procedures:

- Inguinal herniorrhaphy (herniorrhaphy with Marlex mesh is coded to Supplement, not Repair)
- Laparotomy with suture blunt force duodenal laceration
- Perineoplasty with repair of old obstetric laceration
- Suture right biceps tendon laceration

2.85. Closure of skin laceration, left external ear

Code(s): 0HQ3XZZ

2.86. Closure of chest wall stab wound

Code(s): ______________________

2.87. Suture repair of right median nerve laceration, open

Code(s): 01Q50ZZ

Root Operations That Define Other Objectives

Refer to page 491 in the *ICD-10-PCS 2011 Code Book*, Appendix B.

The three root operations belonging to this group are:

- Fusion (G)
- Alteration (0)
- Creation (4)

Fusion – Root Operation G

Fusion G	Definition	Joining together portions of an articular body part rendering the articular body part immobile
	Explanation	The body part is joined together by fixation device, bone graft, or other means
	Examples	Spinal fusion, ankle arthrodesis

A limited range of procedures is represented in the root operation **Fusion**, because fusion procedures are by definition only performed on the joints. Qualifier values are used to specify whether a vertebral joint fusion uses an anterior or posterior approach, and whether the anterior or posterior column of the spine is fused.

Coding Guideline B3.10a. Fusion Procedures of the Spine

The body part coded for a spinal vertebral joint(s) rendered immobile by a spinal fusion procedure is classified by the level of the spine (for example, Thoracic). There are distinct body part values for a single vertebral joint and for multiple joints at each spinal level.

Example: Body part values specify Lumbar Vertebral Joint, Lumbar Vertebral Joints, 2 or More, and Lumbosacral Vertebral Joint.

Coding Guideline B3.10b. Fusion Procedures of the Spine

If multiple vertebral joints are fused, a separate procedure is coded for each vertebral joint that uses a different device and/or qualifier.

Example: Fusion of lumbar vertebral joint, posterior approach, anterior column and fusion of lumbar vertebral joint, posterior approach, posterior column are coded separately.

Coding Guideline B3.10c. Fusion Procedures of the Spine
Combinations of devices and materials are often used on a vertebral joint to render the joint immobile. When combinations of devices are used on the same vertebral joint, the device value coded for the procedure is as follows: If an interbody fusion device is used to render the joint immobile (alone or containing other material like bone graft), the procedure is coded with the device value Interbody Fusions Device; if internal fixation is used to render the joint immobile and an interbody fusion device is *not* used, the procedure is coded with the device value Internal Fixation Device; if bone graft is the *only* device used to render the joint immobile, the procedure is coded with the device value Nonautologous Tissue Substitute or Autologous Tissue Substitute, and if a mixture of autologous and nonautologous bone graft (with or without biological or synthetic extenders or binders) is used to render the joint immobile, code the procedure with the device value Autologous Tissue Substitute.

Examples:

- Fusion of a vertebral joint using a cage style interbody fusion device containing morselized bone graft is coded to the device Interbody Fusion Device.
- Fusion of a vertebral joint using a bone dowel interbody fusion device made of cadaver bone and packed with a mixture of local morselized bone and demineralized bone matrix is coded to the device Interbody Fusion Device.
- Fusion of a vertebral joint using rigid plates affixed with screws and reinforced with bone cement is coded to the device Internal Fixation Device.
- Fusion of a vertebral joint using both autologous bone graft and bone bank bone graft is coded to the device Autologous Tissue substitute.

Additional examples of Fusion procedures:

- Arthrodesis of the right ankle, open
- Intercarpal fusion of left hand with bone bank bone graft, open
- Radiocarpal fusion of right hand with internal fixation, open
- Sacrococcygeal fusion with synthetic substitute, open

Coding Note: When coding fusions, it is important to understand that PCS body part values are classified as joints and not vertebra. For example, if a fusion is done at L1-L2, this is value 0, Lumbar vertebral joint (single), or one joint. If a fusion is done on L1-L3, this is value 1, Lumbar Vertebral Joints, 2 or more, for 2 joints.

2.88. Posterior spinal fusion of the ~~posterior~~ Anterior column at L2-L4 levels with BAK cage interbody fusion device, open

Code(s): 0SG103J

2.89. Interphalangeal fusion of right great toe, percutaneous pin fixation

Code(s): 0SGP34Z

Alteration – Root Operation 0

Alteration 0	Definition	Modifying the natural anatomic structure of a body part without affecting the function of the body part
	Explanation	Principal purpose is to improve appearance
	Examples	Face lift, breast augmentation, cosmetic liposuction (liposuction for medical reasons is Extraction)

Alteration is coded for all procedures performed solely to improve appearance. All methods, approaches, and devices used for the objective of improving appearance are coded here.

Coding Note: Alteration
Because some surgical procedures can be performed for either medical or cosmetic purposes, coding for Alteration requires diagnostic confirmation that the surgery is in fact performed to improve appearance. If the procedure is done for medical conditions, then the appropriate root operation is assigned such as Extraction, Reposition, Resection, Repair, Replacement, and such.

Additional examples of Alteration procedures:

- Abdominal liposuction for cosmetic reasons
- Cosmetic face lift, open
- Cosmetic rhinoplasty with septal reduction and tip elevation, using local tissue graft, open
- Open cosmetic blepharoplasty of right and left lower eyelids

2.90. Abdominoplasty, open (tummy tuck)

Code(s): ______________________________

2.91. Bilateral breast augmentation with silicone implants, open

Code(s): 0H0V0JZ

2.92. Liposuction, bilateral thighs

Code(s): 0J0M3ZZ
0J0L3ZZ

Creation - Root Operation 4 Start by looking up body part

Creation 4	Definition	Making a new genital structure that does not physically take the place of a body part
	Explanation	Used only for sex change operations
	Examples	Creation of vagina in a male, creation of penis in a female

Creation is used to represent a very narrow range of procedures. Only the procedures performed for sex change operations are included here.

Coding Note: Harvesting Autograft Tissue
If a separate procedure is performed to harvest autograft tissue, it is coded to the appropriate root operation in addition to the primary procedure.

The qualifier identifies the body part being created, either vagina or penis. The body part values are M, Perineum, Male or N, Perineum, Female and pertain to the current sex of the patient.

Additional examples of Creation procedures:

- Creation of penis in female patient using synthetic material
- Creation of vagina in male patient using tissue bank donor graft

2.93. Creation of penis in female patient using tissue bank donor graft

Code(s): 0W4N0K1

2.94. Creation of vagina in male patient using synthetic material

Code(s): 0W4M0J0

Part II: ICD-10-PCS Coding

ICD-10-PCS Training – Day 2

Procedures in the Medical and Surgical-related Sections

ICD-10-PCS contains a total of nine Medical and Surgical-related sections as follows:

Section Value	Description
Section 1	Obstetrics
Section 2	Placement
Section 3	Administration
Section 4	Measurement and Monitoring
Section 5	Extracorporeal Assistance and Performance
Section 6	Extracorporeal Therapies
Section 7	Osteopathic
Section 8	Other Procedures
Section 9	Chiropractic

Coding Procedures in the Obstetrics Section – Section 1

Obstetrics Guidelines

C.1 *Products of Conception*
Procedures performed on the products of conception are coded to the Obstetrics section. Procedures performed on the pregnant female other than the products of conception are coded to the appropriate root operation in the Medical and Surgical section.

Example: Amniocentesis is coded to the products of conception body part in the Obstetrics section. Repair of obstetric urethral laceration is coded to the urethra body part in the Medical and Surgical section.

C.2 *Procedures Following Delivery or Abortion*
Procedures performed following a delivery or abortion for curettage of the endometrium or evacuation of retained products of conception are all coded in the Obstetrics section, to the root operation Extraction and the body part Products of Conception, Retained. Diagnostic or therapeutic dilation and curettage performed during times other than the postpartum or post-abortion period are all coded in the Medical and Surgical section, to the root operation Extraction and the body part Endometrium.

Coding Note: Products of Conception

- Products of conception refer to all components of pregnancy, including fetus, embryo, amnion, umbilical cord, and placenta.
- There is no differentiation of the products of conception based on gestational age.

Characters of Obstetrics Section

The seven characters in the Obstetrics section are:

Character 1 Section	Character 2 Body System	Character 3 Root Operation	Character 4 Body Part	Character 5 Approach	Character 6 Device	Character 7 Qualifier

The **Obstetrics** section follows the same conventions established in the Medical and Surgical section, with all seven characters retaining the same meaning.

Character 2 (Body System) – one single body system, **Pregnancy**

Character 4 (Body Part) – three body part values:

- Products of conception
- Products of conception, retained
- Products of conception, ectopic

Root Operations in Obstetrics Section

Refer to page 485 in the *ICD-10-PCS 2011 Code Book*, Appendix A.

There are a total of 12 root operations in the Obstetrics section; 10 of the root operations are found in other sections of ICD-10-PCS and two are unique to the Obstetrics section. The two unique root operations to the Obstetrics section are **Abortion** and **Delivery**.

Obstetrics Section Root Operations			
Abortion	Change	***Delivery***	Drainage
Extraction	Insertion	Inspection	Removal
Repair	Reposition	Resection	Transplantation

Obstetrics Section Qualifier

The qualifier values are dependent upon the root operation, approach, or body system.

Examples:

- Methods of extraction – low forceps, vacuum, low cervical
- Methods of terminating pregnancy – laminaria, abortifacient
- Substances drained – amniotic fluid, fetal cerebrospinal fluid

Abortion – Root Operation A

Abortion A	Definition	Artificially terminating a pregnancy
	Explanation	Subdivided according to whether an additional device such as a laminaria or abortifacient is used; or whether the abortion was performed by mechanical means
	Examples	Transvaginal abortion using vacuum aspiration technique

Abortion is subdivided according to whether an additional device such as a laminaria or abortifacient is used, or whether the abortion was performed by mechanical means. If either a laminaria or abortifacient is used, then the approach is via natural or artificial opening. All other abortion procedures are those done by mechanical means (the products of conception are physically removed using instrumentation) and the device value is Z, no device.

3.1. Transvaginal abortion using vacuum aspiration technique

Code(s): 10A07Z6

Delivery – Root Operation E

Delivery E	Definition	Assisting the passage of the products of conception from the genital canal
	Explanation	Applies only to manually assisted, vaginal delivery
	Example	Manually assisted delivery

Delivery applies only to manually assisted, vaginal delivery and is defined as assisting the passage of products of conception from the genital canal. Cesarean deliveries are coded in this section to the root operation Extraction.

3.2. Manually assisted delivery

Code(s): 10E0XZZ

Drainage – Root Operation 9

Drainage 9	Definition	Taking or letting out fluids and/or gases from a body part
	Explanation	The qualifier identifies the substance that is drained from the products of conception (fetal blood, fetal spinal fluid, amniotic fluid).
	Examples	Amniocentesis, percutaneous fetal spinal tap

The root operation **Drainage** is coded for both diagnostic and therapeutic drainage procedures. For the Obstetrics section the qualifier values identify the substance that is drained from the products of conception (for example, fetal blood, amniotic fluid).

3.3. Fetal spinal tap, percutaneous

Code(s): ~~10E0XZZ~~ 10903ZA

Coding Procedures in the Placement Section – Section 2

Characters of Placement Section

The seven characters in the Placement section are:

Character 1 Section	Character 2 Body System	Character 3 Root Operation	Character 4 Body Region	Character 5 Approach	Character 6 Device	Character 7 Qualifier

The **Placement** section follows the same conventions established in the Medical and Surgical section, with all seven characters retaining the same meaning.

Character 2 (Body System) – two body system values

- Anatomical Regions
- Anatomical Orifices

Character 4 (Body Region) – two body region types

- External body regions (for example, chest wall)
- Natural orifices (for example, mouth and pharynx)

Root Operations in Placement Section

Refer to pages 485-486 in the *ICD-10-PCS 2011 Code Book*, Appendix A.

The root operations in the **Placement** section include only those procedures performed without making an incision or puncture. There are a total of seven root operations in the **Placement** section of which two are common to other sections—**Change** and **Removal**. The five additional root operations unique to the **Placement** section are **Compression, Dressing, Immobilization, Packing,** and **Traction**.

Placement Section Root Operations			
Change	***Compression***	***Dressing***	***Immobilization***
Packing	Removal	***Traction***	

Devices in Placement Section

- Specifies the material or device in placement procedure (for example, splint, traction apparatus, pressure dressing, bandage)
- Includes casts for fractures and dislocations
- Devices in the Placement section are off the shelf and do not require any extensive design, fabrication, or fitting
- The placement of devices that require extensive design, fabrication, or fitting are coded in the Rehabilitation section of ICD-10-PCS

Packing – Root Operation 4

Packing 4	Definition	Putting material in a body region or orifice
	Explanation	Procedures performed without making an incision or puncture
	Example	Placement of nasal packing

3.4. Placement of nasal packing

Code(s): 2Y41X5Z

Immobilization – Root Operation 3

Immobilization 3	Definition	Limiting or preventing motion of a body region
	Explanation	Procedures to fit a device, such as splints or braces, apply only to the rehabilitation setting
	Example	Placement of splint on left finger

Coding Note: Immobilization
The procedures to fit a device, such as splints and braces as described in F0DZ6EZ and F0DZ7EZ, apply only to the rehabilitation setting. Splints and braces placed in other inpatient settings are coded to **Immobilization**, Table 2W3 in the **Placement** section.

3.5. Placement of splint, left hand

Code(s): 2W3FX1Z

Compression – Root Operation 1

Compression 1	Definition	Putting pressure on a body region
	Explanation	Procedures performed without making an incision or puncture
	Example	Placement of pressure dressing on abdominal wall

3.6. Placement of intermittent pneumatic compression device, covering left lower leg

Code(s): ______

Dressing – Root Operation 2

Dressing 2	Definition	Putting material on a body region for protection
	Explanation	Procedures performed without making an incision or puncture
	Example	Application of sterile dressing to head wound

3.7. Sterile dressing placement to wound of the chest wall

Code(s): ____

Traction – Root Operation 6

Traction 6	Definition	Exerting a pulling force on a body region in a distal direction
	Explanation	Traction in this section includes only the task performed using a mechanical traction apparatus
	Example	Lumbar traction using motorized split-traction table

Traction in this section includes only the task performed using a mechanical traction apparatus. Manual traction performed by a physical therapist is coded to Manual Therapy Techniques in section F, Physical Rehabilitation and Diagnostic Audiology.

3.8. Mechanical traction of entire right leg

Code(s): ____

Coding Procedures in the Administration Section – Section 3

Characters of Administration Section

The seven characters in the Administration section are:

Character 1 Section	Character 2 Body System	Character 3 Root Operation	Character 4 Body System/ Region	Character 5 Approach	Character 6 Substance	Character 7 Qualifier

Character 2 (Body System) – three body system values

- Physiological Systems and Anatomical Regions
- Circulatory
- Indwelling Device

Character 5 (Approach)

- Uses values defined in the Medical and Surgical section
- The approach value for intradermal, subcutaneous, and intramuscular introduction (that is, injections) is percutaneous
- If a catheter is used to introduce a substance into a site within the circulatory system, the approach value is percutaneous

Character 6 (Substance)

- Substances are specified in broad categories
- Substance values depend on body part

Root Operations in Administration Section

Refer to page 486 in the *ICD-10-PCS 2011 Code Book*, Appendix A.

The root operations in this section are classified according to the broad category of substance administered. If the substance given is a blood product or a cleansing substance, then the procedure is coded to **Transfusion** and **Irrigation** respectively. All other substances administered, such as antineoplastic substances, are coded to the root operation, **Introduction**.

Administration Section Root Operations		
Introduction	***Irrigation***	***Transfusion***

Substances in Administrative Section

Character 6 in the Administrative section specifies the substances given and broad categories are specified with the substance values dependent on the body part.

Administrative Section Substances Physiological Systems and Anatomical Regions			
Anti-inflammatory	Anti-infective	Antineoplastic	Antiarrhythmic
Dialysate	Electrolytic and Water Balance Substance	Gas	Intracirculatory Anesthetic
Local Anesthetic	Nutritional Substance	Pancreatic Islet Cells	Pigment
Platelet Inhibitor	Radioactive Substance	Regional Anesthetic	Serum, Toxoid, and Vaccine
Sperm	Stem Cells, Embryonic	Stem Cells, Somatic	Thrombolytic

Administrative Section Substances Circulatory			
Antihemolytic factor	Bone Marrow	Factor IX	Fibrinogen
Fresh Plasma	Frozen Plasma	Globulin	Platelets
Red Blood Cells	Frozen Red Cells	Serum Albumin	Whole Blood

Coding Note: Administration Section
The **Administration** section includes infusions, injections, and transfusions, as well as other related procedures, such as irrigation and tattooing. All codes in this section define procedures where a diagnostic or therapeutic substance is given to the patient.

Transfusion – Root Operation 2

Transfusion 2	Definition	Putting in blood or blood products
	Explanation	Substance given is a blood product or a stem cell substance
	Example	Transfusion of cell saver red cells into central venous line

Substance TRANSfusion
3.9. Bone marrow transplant using donor marrow from identical twin, central vein infusion

Code(s): 30243G1

3.10. Transfusion of cell saver red cells via central venous catheter

Code(s): ______

Irrigation – Root Operation 1

Irrigation 1	Definition	Putting in or on a cleansing substance
	Explanation	Substance given is a cleansing substance or dialysate
	Example	Flushing of eye

Coding Note: Body Part Value
For the root operation Irrigation, the body part value specifies the site of the irrigation.

3.11. Peritoneal dialysis via indwelling catheter

Code(s): 3E1M39Z

3.12. Percutaneous irrigation of knee joint

Code(s): ______________________________

Introduction – Root Operation 0

Introduction 0	Definition	Putting in or on a therapeutic, diagnostic, nutritional, physiological, or prophylactic substance except blood or blood products
	Explanation	All other substances administered, such as antineoplastic substance
	Example	Nerve block injection to median nerve

Coding Note: Substance for Mixed Steroid and Local Anesthetic
When a substance of mixed steroid and local anesthetic is given for pain control it is coded to the substance value **Anti-Inflammatory**. The anesthetic is only added to lessen the pain of the injection.

Coding Note: Body Part Value
For the root operation Introduction, the body part value specifies where the procedure occurs and not necessarily the site where the substance introduced has an effect.

3.13. Lumbar epidural injection of mixed steroid and local anesthetic for pain control

Code(s): ______________________________

Coding Procedures in the Measurement and Monitoring Section – Section 4

Characters of Measurement and Monitoring Section

The seven characters in the Measurement and Monitoring section are:

Character 1 Section	Character 2 Body System	Character 3 Root Operation	Character 4 Body System	Character 5 Approach	Character 6 Function/ Device	Character 7 Qualifier

Character 2 (Body System) – two body system values, **Physiological Systems and Physiological Devices (Note: Physiological Devices is a body system value for Measurement only)**

Character 6 (Function/Device) – specifies physiological or physical function being tested (for example, nerve conductivity, respiratory capacity)

Root Operations in Measurement and Monitoring Section

Refer to page 486 in the *ICD-10-PCS 2011 Code Book*, Appendix A.

There are only two root operations in the **Measurement and Monitoring** section. **Measurement** is the first root operation and is used when the procedure determines the level of a physiological or physical function at a point in time. **Monitoring** is the second root operation and is used when the procedure determines the level of a physiological or physical function repetitively over a period of time.

Measurement and Monitoring Section Root Operations	
Measurement	***Monitoring***

Measurement – Root Operation 0

Measurement 0	Definition	Determining the level of a physiological or physical function at a point in time
	Explanation	A single temperature reading is considered a measurement
	Example	External EKG, single reading

3.14. Left heart catheterization with sampling and pressure measurements

Code(s): 4A023N7

Monitoring – Root Operation 1

Monitoring 1	Definition	Determining the level of a physiological or physical function repetitively over a period of time
	Explanation	Temperature taken every half hour for 8 hours is considered monitoring
	Example	Urinary pressure monitoring

3.15. Ambulatory Holter monitoring

Code(s): ______________________________

3.16. Transvaginal fetal heart rate monitoring over a period of 16 hours

Code(s): 4A1H7CZ

Coding Procedures in the Extracorporeal Assistance and Performance Section – Section 5

Characters of Extracorporeal Assistance and Performance Section

The seven characters in the Extracorporeal Assistance and Performance section are:

Character 1 Section	Character 2 Body System	Character 3 Root Operation	Character 4 Body System	Character 5 Duration	Character 6 Function	Character 7 Qualifier

Character 2 (Body System) – single body system value, **Physiological Systems**

Character 5 (Duration) – specifies whether the procedure was a single occurrence, multiple occurrence, intermittent, or continuous

Character 6 (Function) – specifies the physiological function assisted or performed (for example, oxygenation, ventilation)

Coding Note: Character 5 – Duration
For respiratory ventilation assistance or performance, the range of consecutive hours is specified (<24 hours, 24–96 hours, or >96 hours).

Root Operation in Extracorporeal Assistance and Performance Section

Refer to page 486 in the *ICD-10-PCS 2011 Code Book*, Appendix A.

There are three unique root operations in the **Extracorporeal Assistance and Performance** section: **Assistance, Performance,** and **Restoration. Assistance** and **Performance** are two variations of the same kinds of procedures, varying only in the degree of control exercised over the physiological function. **Assistance** is taking over partial control of the physiological function and **Performance** is taking complete control of the physiological function. **Restoration** is returning a physiological function to its original state.

Extracorporeal Assistance and Performance Section Root Operations		
Assistance	***Performance***	***Restoration***

Assistance – Root Operation 0

Assistance 0	Definition	Taking over a portion of a physiological function by extracorporeal means
	Explanation	Procedures that support a physiological function but do not take complete control of it, such as intra-aortic balloon pump to support cardiac output and hyperbaric oxygen treatment
	Example	Hyperbaric oxygenation of wound

3.17. Intra-aortic balloon pump (IABP), continuous

Code(s): ______________________________

Performance – Root Operation 1

Performance 1	Definition	Completely taking over a physiological function by extracorporeal means
	Explanation	Procedures in which complete control is exercised over a physiological function, such as total mechanical ventilation, cardiac pacing, and cardiopulmonary bypass
	Example	Cardiopulmonary bypass in conjunction with CABG

3.18. Hemodialysis, single encounter

Code(s): ____________________

3.19. Cardiopulmonary bypass with CABG, 8 hours

Code(s): 5A1221Z 5A1935Z
Cardiac Output Respiratory Vent.

Restoration – Root Operation 2

Restoration 2	Definition	Returning, or attempting to return, a physiological function to its original state by extracorporeal means
	Explanation	Restoration defines only external cardioversion and defibrillation procedures. Failed cardioversion procedures are also included in the definition of Restoration and are coded the same as successful procedures.
	Example	Attempted cardiac defibrillation, unsuccessful

3.20. External cardioversion

Code(s): ~~5A1221Z~~

Coding Procedures in the Extracorporeal Therapies Section – Section 6

Characters of Extracorporeal Therapies Section

The seven characters in the Extracorporeal Therapies section are:

Character 1 Section	Character 2 Body System	Character 3 Root Operation	Character 4 Body System	Character 5 Duration	Character 6 Qualifier	Character 7 Qualifier

Character 2 (Body System) – single body system value, **Physiological Systems**

Character 5 (Duration) – specifies whether the procedure was single occurrence, multiple occurrence or intermittent

Character 6 (Qualifier) – no specific qualifier values (Z – no qualifier)

Character 7 (Qualifier) – identifies various blood components separated out in pheresis procedures

Root Operation in Extracorporeal Therapies Section

Refer to page 487 in the *ICD-10-PCS 2011 Code Book*, Appendix A.

There are 10 root operations within the **Extracorporeal Therapies** section and the meaning of each root operation is consistent with the term as used in the medical community.

- **Atmospheric Control (value 0)** – extracorporeal control of atmospheric pressure and composition
- **Decompression (value1)** – extracorporeal elimination of undissolved gas from body fluids
- **Electromagnetic Therapy (value 2)** – extracorporeal treatment by electromagnetic rays
- **Hyperthermia (value 3)** – extracorporeal raising of the body temperature
- **Hypothermia (value 4)** – extracorporeal lowering of the body temperature
- **Pheresis (value 5)** – extracorporeal separation of blood products
- **Phototherapy (value 6)** – extracorporeal treatment by light rays
- **Ultrasound Therapy (value 7)** – extracorporeal treatment by ultrasound
- **Ultraviolet Light Therapy (value 8)** – extracorporeal treatment by ultraviolet lights
- **Shock Wave Therapy (value 9)** – extracorporeal treatment by shock waves

Extracorporeal Therapies Section Root Operations			
Atmospheric Control	***Decompression***	***Electromagnetic Therapy***	***Hyperthermia***
Hypothermia	***Pheresis***	***Phototherapy***	***Ultrasound Therapy***
Ultraviolet Light Therapy	***Shock Wave Therapy***		

Coding Note: Decompression
Decompression describes a single type of procedure – treatment for decompression sickness (the bends) in a hyperbaric chamber.

Coding Note: Hyperthermia
Hyperthermia is used both to treat temperature imbalance, and as an adjunct radiation treatment for cancer. When performed to treat temperature imbalance, the procedure is coded to this section.

When performed for cancer treatment, whole-body hyperthermia is classified as a modality qualifier in section D, Radiation Oncology.

Coding Note: Pheresis
Pheresis is used in medical practice for two main purposes: to treat diseases where too much of a blood component is produced, such as leukemia, or to remove a blood product such as platelets from a donor, for transfusion into a patient who needs them.

Coding Note: Phototherapy
Phototherapy to the circulatory system means exposing the blood to light rays outside the body, using a machine that recirculates the blood and returns it to the body after phototherapy.

3.21. Whole body hypothermia, single treatment (for treatment of temperature imbalance)

Code(s): ______________________________

3.22. Ultraviolet light phototherapy, single treatment

Code(s): ______________________________

Coding Procedures in the Osteopathic Section – Section 7

Characters of Osteopathic Section

The seven characters in the Osteopathic section are:

Character 1 Section	Character 2 Body System	Character 3 Root Operation	Character 4 Body Region	Character 5 Approach	Character 6 Method	Character 7 Qualifier

Character 2 (Body System) – single body system value, **Anatomical Regions**

Character 6 (Method) – method of the osteopathic treatment; these methods are not explicitly defined in ICD-10-PCS and rely on the standard definitions as used in this specialty.

Root Operation in Osteopathic Section

Refer to page 487 in the *ICD-10-PCS 2011 Code Book*, Appendix A.

The Osteopathic section contains a single root operation, **Treatment**.

Osteopathic Methods

Character 6 in the Osteopathic section defines the osteopathic method of the procedure.

Osteopathic Methods			
Articulatory – Raising	Fascial Release	General Mobilization	High Velocity – Low Amplitude
Indirect	Low Velocity – High Amplitude	Lymphatic Pump	Muscle Energy – Isometric
Muscle Energy – Isotonic	Other Method		

Coding Note: Osteopathic Section
Section 7, Osteopathic, is one of the smallest sections in ICD-10-PCS. There is a single body system, **Anatomic Regions**, and a single root operation, **Treatment**.

Treatment – Root Operation 0

Treatment 0	Definition	Manual treatment to eliminate or alleviate somatic dysfunction and related disorder
	Explanation	None
	Example	Fascial release of abdomen, osteopathic treatment

3.23. Indirect osteopathic treatment of sacrum

Code(s): ______________________________

Coding Procedures in the Other Procedures Section – Section 8

Characters of Other Procedures Section

The seven characters in the Other Procedures section are:

Character 1 Section	Character 2 Body System	Character 3 Root Operation	Character 4 Body Region	Character 5 Approach	Character 6 Method	Character 7 Qualifier

Character 2 (Body System) – two body system values, Indwelling Device and Physiological Systems and Anatomical Regions

Character 6 (Method) – defines the method of the procedure, such as robotic assisted procedure, computer-assisted procedure, or acupuncture

Root Operation in Other Procedures Section

Refer to page 487 in the *ICD-10-PCS 2011 Code Book*, Appendix A.

The Other Procedures section contains a single root operation, **Other Procedures**.

> **Coding Note: Other Procedures Section**
> The Other Procedures section contains codes for procedures not included in the other Medical and Surgical-related sections. There are relatively few procedures coded in this section. Whole body therapies including acupuncture and meditation are included in this section along with a code for the fertilization portion of an in-vitro fertilization procedure. This section also contains codes for robotic assisted and computer assisted procedures.

Other Procedures – Root Operation 0

Other Procedures 0	Definition	Methodologies that attempt to remediate or cure a disorder or disease
	Explanation	For nontraditional, whole-body therapies including acupuncture and meditation
	Example	Acupuncture

3.24. Robotic-assisted transurethral prostatectomy

Code(s): ~~8E08CZ~~ 8E0W8CZ

3.25. Suture removal, right leg

Code(s): ______________________

Coding Procedures in the Chiropractic Section – Section 9

Characters of Chiropractic Section

The seven characters in the Chiropractic section are:

Character 1 Section	Character 2 Body System	Character 3 Root Operation	Character 4 Body Region	Character 5 Approach	Character 6 Method	Character 7 Qualifier

Character 2 (Body System) – single body system value, **Anatomical Regions**

Root Operation in Chiropractic Section

Refer to page 488 in the *ICD-10-PCS 2011 Code Book*, Appendix A.

The Chiropractic Section contains a single root operation, **Manipulation**.

Coding Note: Chiropractic Section Section 9, Chiropractic section, consists of a single body system, **Anatomical Regions**, and a single root operation, **Manipulation**.

Manipulation – Root Operation B

Manipulation B	Definition	Manual procedures that involves a direct thrust to move a joint past the physiological range of motion, without exceeding the anatomical limit
	Explanation	None
	Example	Chiropractic treatment of cervical spine, short lever specific contact

3.26. Chiropractic treatment of lumbar spine using long and short lever specific contact

Code(s): ______________________________

Procedures in the Ancillary Sections

ICD-10-PCS contains a total of six ancillary sections as follows:

Section Value	**Description**
Section B	Imaging
Section C	Nuclear Medicine
Section D	Radiation Oncology
Section F	Physical Rehabilitation and Diagnostic Audiology
Section G	Mental Health
Section H	Substance Abuse Treatment

Note: Ancillary sections (sections B–D and F–H) do not include root operations. Character 3 represents root type of the procedure for these sections.

Coding Procedures in the Imaging Section – Section B

Characters of Imaging Section

The seven characters in the Imaging section are:

Character 1 Section	Character 2 Body System	Character 3 Root Type	Character 4 Body Part	Character 5 Contrast	Character 6 Qualifier	Character 7 Qualifier

Character 3 (Root Type) – defines procedure by root type, instead of root operation

Character 5 (Contrast) – defines contrast if used; contrast is differentiated by the concentration of the contrast material (for example, high or low osmolar)

Character 6 (Qualifier) – for majority of imaging codes is a qualifier that specifies an image is taken without contrast followed by one with contrast (unenhanced and enhanced (0)); occasionally also specifies laser (1) or intravascular optical coherence (2)

Character 7 (Qualifier) – for majority of imaging codes is a qualifier that is not specified in this section; occasionally specifies intraoperative (0), densitometry (1), intravascular (3), transesophageal (4), or guidance (A)

Root Types in Imaging Section

The Imaging section has a total of five root types:

- Plain Radiography (value 0) – Planar display of an image developed from the capture of external ionizing radiation on photographic or photoconductive plate
- Fluoroscopy (value 1) – Single plane or bi-plane real time display of an image developed from the capture of external ionizing radiation on a fluorescent screen. The image may also be stored by either digital or analog means.

- Computerized Tomography (CT scan) (value 2) – Computer reformatted digital display of multiplanar images developed from the capture of multiple exposures of external ionizing radiation
- Magnetic Resonance Imaging (MRI) (value 3) – Computer reformatted digital display of multiplanar images developed from the capture of radio-frequency signals emitted by nuclei in a body site excited within a magnetic field
- Ultrasonography (value 4) – Real time display of images of anatomy or flow information developed from the capture of reflected and attenuated high frequency sound waves

3.27. MRI of thyroid gland, without contrast material followed by with other contrast material

Code(s): ______________________________

3.28. Chest x-ray, anteroposterior (AP) and posteroanterior (PA)

Code(s): ______________________________

Coding Procedures in the Nuclear Medicine Section – Section C

Characters of Nuclear Medicine Section

The seven characters in the Nuclear Medicine section are:

Character 1 Section	Character 2 Body System	Character 3 Root Type	Character 4 Body Part	Character 5 Radionuclide	Character 6 Qualifier	Character 7 Qualifier

Character 3 (Root Type) – defines procedure by root type, instead of root operation

Character 5 (Radionuclide) – defines the source of the radiation used in the procedure; an "Other Radionuclide" option is included for new FDA radiopharmaceuticals

Characters 6 and 7 (Qualifiers) – are not specified in this section (Z)

Root Types in Nuclear Medicine Section

The Nuclear Medicine section has a total of seven root types:

- Planar Nuclear Medicine Imaging (value 1) – Introduction of radioactive materials into the body for single plane display of images developed from the capture of radioactive emissions
- Tomographic (Tomo) Nuclear Medicine Imaging (value 2) – Introduction of radioactive materials into the body for three-dimensional display of images developed from the capture of radioactive emissions
- Positron Emission Tomography (PET) (value 3) – Introduction of radioactive materials into the body for three-dimensional display of images developed from the simultaneous capture, 180 degrees apart, of radioactive emissions
- Nonimaging Nuclear Medicine Uptake (value 4) – Introduction of radioactive materials into the body for measurements of organ function, from the detection of radioactive emissions
- Nonimaging Nuclear Medicine Probe (value 5) – Introduction of radioactive materials into the body for the study of distribution and fate of certain substances by the detection of radioactive emissions from an external source
- Nonimaging Nuclear Medicine Assay (value 6) – Introduction of radioactive materials into the body for the study of body fluids and blood elements, by the detection of radioactive emissions
- Systemic Nuclear Medicine Therapy (value 7) – Introduction of unsealed radioactive materials into the body for treatment

3.29. PET scan of myocardium using Fluorine 18 (F-18)

Code(s): ____

3.30. Technetium tomo scan of the spleen

Code(s): ____

Coding Procedures in the Radiation Oncology Section – Section D

Characters of Radiation Oncology Section

The seven characters in the Radiation Oncology section are:

Character 1 Section	Character 2 Body System	Character 3 Root Type	Character 4 Treatment Site	Character 5 Modality Qualifier	Character 6 Isotope	Character 7 Qualifier

Character 3 (Root Type) – specifies the basic modality (beam radiation, brachytherapy, stereotactic radiosurgery, and other radiation)

Character 4 (Treatment Site) – specifies the treatment site that is the target of the radiation therapy

Character 5 (Modality Qualifier) – further specifies treatment modality (photons, electrons, heavy particles, contact radiation)

Character 6 (Isotope) – specifies the radioactive isotope administered in the oncology treatment

3.31. Brachytherapy of prostate, HDR using Cesium 137

Code(s): DV10972

3.32. Contact radiation of esophagus

Code(s): ______

Coding Procedures in the Physical Rehabilitation and Diagnostic Audiology Section – Section F

Characters of Physical Rehabilitation and Diagnostic Audiology Section

The seven characters in the Physical Rehabilitation and Diagnostic Audiology section are:

Character 1 Section	Character 2 Section Qualifier	Character 3 Root Type	Character 4 Body System/ Region	Character 5 Type Qualifier	Character 6 Equipment	Character 7 Qualifier

Character 2 (Section Qualifier) – specifies whether the procedure is a rehabilitation or diagnostic audiology procedure

Character 3 (Root Type) – specifies general procedure root type

Character 4 (Body System/Region) – specifies the body system and body region combined, where applicable

Character 5 (Type Qualifier) – specifies the precise test or method employed (Refer to pages 513--520 in the *ICD-10-PCS 2011 Code Book*, Appendix D, for Type Qualifier Definitions.)

Character 6 (Equipment) – specifies the general categories of equipment used, if any (Note: specific types of equipment are not listed.)

Root Types in Physical Rehabilitation and Diagnostic Audiology Section

The Physical Rehabilitation and Diagnostic Audiology section classifies procedures into 14 root types:

- Speech Assessment (value 0) – Measurement of speech and related functions
- Motor and/or Nerve Function Assessment (value 1) – Measurement of motor, nerve, and related functions
- Activities of Daily Living Assessment (value 2) – Measurement of functional level for activities of daily living
- Hearing Assessment (value 3) – Measurement of hearing and related functions
- Hearing Aid Assessment (value 4) – Measurement of the appropriateness and/or effectiveness of a hearing device
- Vestibular Assessment (value 5) – Measurement of the vestibular system and related functions
- Speech Treatment (value 6) – Application of techniques to improve, augment, or compensate for speech and related functional impairment
- Motor Treatment (value 7) – Exercise or activities to increase or facilitate motor function

- Activities of Daily Living Treatment (value 8) – Exercise or activities to facilitate functional competence for activities of daily living
- Hearing Treatment (value 9) – Application of techniques to improve, augment, or compensate for hearing and related functional impairment
- Hearing Aid Treatment (value B) – Application of techniques to improve the communication abilities of individuals with cochlear implant
- Vestibular Treatment (value C) – Application of techniques to improve, augment, or compensate for vestibular and related functional impairment
- Device Fitting (value D) – Fitting of a device designed to facilitate or support achievement of a higher level of function
- Caregiver Training (value F) – Training in activities to support patient's optimal level of function

Coding Note: Treatment
Use of specific activities or methods to develop, improve and/or restore the performance of necessary functions, compensate for dysfunction and/or minimize debilitation.

Treatment procedures include swallowing dysfunction exercises, bathing and showering techniques, wound management, gait training, and a host of activities typically associated with rehabilitation.

Coding Note: Assessment
Assessment includes a determination of the patient's diagnosis when appropriate, need for treatment, planning for treatment, periodic assessment and documentation related to these activities.

Assessments are further classified into more than 100 different tests or methods. The majority of these focus on the faculties of hearing and speech, but others focus on various aspects of body function, and on the patient's quality of life, such as muscle performance, neuromotor development, and reintegration skills.

Coding Note: Device Fitting
Design, fabrication, modification, selection and/or application of splint, orthosis, prosthesis, hearing aids and/or rehabilitation device. Device Fitting describes the device being fitted rather than the method used to fit the device.

Coding Note: Caregiver Training
Educating caregiver with the skills and knowledge used to interact with and assist the patient. Caregiver Training is divided into 18 different broad subjects taught to help a caregiver provide proper patient care.

3.33. Wound care treatment of right lower leg ulcer (staged to muscle) using pulsatile lavage

Code(s): ______________________________

3.34. Bekesy assessment using audiometer

Code(s): ______________________________

Coding Procedures in the Mental Health Section – Section G

Characters of Mental Health Section

The seven characters in the Mental Health section are:

Character 1 Section	Character 2 Body System	Character 3 Root Type	Character 4 Type Qualifier	Character 5 Qualifier	Character 6 Qualifier	Character 7 Qualifier

Character 2 (Body System) – does not convey specific information about the procedure, the value Z functions as a placeholder for this character

Character 3 (Root Type) – specifies the mental health procedure root type

Character 4 (Type Qualifier) – further specifies the procedure type as needed

Characters 5, 6, and 7 (Qualifier) – do not convey specific information about the procedure, the value Z functions as a placeholder for these characters

Root Types in Mental Health Section

There are 11 root type values in the Mental Health section:

- Psychological Tests – value 1
- Crisis Intervention – value 2
- Individual Psychotherapy – value 5
- Counseling – value 6
- Family Psychotherapy – value 7
- Electroconvulsive Therapy – value B
- Biofeedback – value C
- Hypnosis – value F
- Narcosynthesis – value G
- Group Therapy – value H
- Light Therapy – value J

3.35. Electroconvulsive therapy (ECT), bilateral, multiple seizures

Code(s): GZB3ZZZ

3.36. Personality and Behavioral Testing

Code(s): ______________________

Coding Procedures in the Substance Abuse Treatment Section – Section H

Characters of Substance Abuse Treatment Section

The seven characters in the Substance Abuse Treatment section are:

Character 1 Section	Character 2 Body System	Character 3 Root Type	Character 4 Type Qualifier	Character 5 Qualifier	Character 6 Qualifier	Character 7 Qualifier

Character 2 (Body System) – does not convey specific information about the procedure, the value Z functions as a placeholder for this character

Character 3 (Root Type) – specifies the root type

Character 4 (Type Qualifier) – further classifies the root type

Characters 5, 6, and 7 (Qualifier) – do not convey specific information about the procedure, the value Z functions as a placeholder for these characters

Root Types in Substance Abuse Treatment Section

There are seven different root type values in the Substance Abuse Treatment section:

- Detoxification Services – value 2
- Individual Counseling – value 3
- Group Counseling – value 4
- Individual Psychotherapy – value 5
- Family Counseling – value 6
- Medication Management – value 8
- Pharmacotherapy – value 9

3.37. Alcohol detoxification treatment

Code(s): HZ2ZZZZ

3.38. Individual 12-step psychotherapy for substance abuse

Code(s): ____________________

Case Studies from Inpatient Health Records

Detailed and/or Complex Cases and Scenarios Using ICD-10-PCS Procedure Codes

Coding Guideline B3.2a. Multiple Procedures
During the same operative episode, multiple procedures are coded if the same root operation is performed on different body parts as defined by distinct values of the body part character.

Coding Guideline B4.3. Bilateral Body Part Values
Bilateral body part values are available for a limited number of body parts. If the identical procedure is performed on contralateral body parts, and a bilateral body part value exists for that body part, a single procedure is coded using the bilateral body part value. If no bilateral body part value exists, each procedure is coded separately using the appropriate body part value.

3.39.
Preoperative Diagnosis: Abnormal bleeding; pelvic pain; uterine retroversion and malposition; uterine descensus; abnormal liver function studies; status-postop ovarian cystectomies; status-postop cesarean section, tubal ligation

Postoperative Diagnosis: Same

Operation: Total abdominal hysterectomy; bilateral salpingo-oophorectomy; liver biopsy

Procedure: With the patient in the supine position under general anesthesia, the abdomen was prepped and draped in the usual sterile fashion. A Pfannenstiel incision was made in the area of the patient's previous Pfannenstiel incision and this was carried down through the subcutaneous fat to the fascia, which was incised transversely. The fascia was dissected off of the underlying rectus muscles. Bleeders were coagulated. The rectus muscles were separated from the fascia above. There was some scarring of the fascia, particularly on the patient's left side. The rectus muscles were parted. The peritoneum was identified. Entry was made into the peritoneal cavity without difficulty. The peritoneal incision was carried inferiorly to superiorly. At this point, I explored the upper abdomen and performed a Tru-Cut needle biopsy of the left lobe of the liver without difficulty.

Coagulation was utilized to control bleeding. Hemostasis was established and at the end of the procedure, the area of the biopsy site was re-evaluated and was noted to be hemostatic. A moist lap was used against this area for compression during the remaining portion of the case, and this lap was removed prior to closing the abdomen.

At this time, the O'Conner-O'Sullivan retractor was put in place. A series of moist laps were used to pack the bowel out of the operative field. The uterus was noted to be markedly retroverted with marked pelvic congestion and the large infundibulopelvic vessels were noted, as well as the broad ligament. The round ligaments were bilaterally doubly Heaney clamped, cut, and suture ligated with 0 Vicryl. The anterior leaf of the broad ligament and posterior leaf of the broad ligament were sharply dissected. Hemostasis was accomplished by coagulation. The quadrangular space was bluntly penetrated bilaterally. Two ligatures of 0 Vicryl were put in place along the infundibulopelvic vessels after taking care to assure the location of the ureters was out of the operative field. This area was then clamped and cut. Hemostasis along the infundibulopelvic pedicle was noted to be good. The ovaries and fallopian tubes were bilaterally removed. There was a right ovarian cyst with multiple smaller cysts noted on the right ovary. The left ovary appeared to be somewhat scarred and was small and reflective of a previous partial oophorectomy, which was performed many years ago on this ovary. The anterior leaf of the broad ligament was sharply dissected. The bladder was sharply dissected off the anterior aspect of the lower uterine segment.

The uterine vessels were bilaterally doubly Heaney clamped, cut, and suture ligated with 0 Vicryl. The remaining portions of the uterine vessels and cardinal ligaments were singularly Ochsner clamped, cut, and suture ligated with 0 Vicryl. The bladder was further dissected off of the anterior aspect of the lower uterine segment. The uterosacral ligaments were singularly Ochsner clamped, cut, and suture ligated with 0 Vicryl, which was held. Entrance was made into the lateral aspects of the vagina. The cervix was sharply dissected away from the vaginal mucosa and noted to be intact in its removal. Aldrich angle sutures were put in place bilaterally. The anterior and posterior vaginal cuffs were approximated with a series of interrupted figure-of-eight sutures utilizing 0 Vicryl. Hemostasis was noted to be good. Copious irrigation was carried out with good evidence of hemostasis in the pelvis. At this time, the O'Conner-O'Sullivan and lap squares were removed. Further visualization of the liver biopsy site was noted and found to be hemostatic.

At this point, the abdomen was closed in a series of layers. The peritoneum was closed with 0 Vicryl in a running fashion. The rectus muscles were reapproximated with 0 Vicryl interrupted mattress sutures. The fascia was closed with #1 Vicryl in a running fashion. Small bleeders were coagulated in the subcutaneous fat. The skin was closed with staples. A sterile dressing was applied. The patient will be sent to Recovery following the procedure. Sponge, lap, and instrument counts were correct times two.

Code(s): 0UT90ZZ 0UTC0ZZ 0UT20ZZ 0UT70ZZ 0FB20ZX

> **Coding Guideline B3.15. Reposition for Fracture Treatment**
> Reduction of a displaced fracture is coded to the root operation Reposition and the application of a cast or splint in conjunction with the Reposition procedure is not coded separately. Treatment of a nondisplaced fracture is coded to the procedure performed.

> **Coding Guideline B4.7. Fingers and Toes**
> If a body system does not contain a separate body part value for fingers, procedures performed on the fingers are coded to the body part value for the hand. If a body system does not contain a separate body part value for toes, procedures performed on the toes are coded to the body part value for the foot.

3.40.

Preoperative Diagnosis: Extensive laceration of distal left index finger with partial severance of distal phalanx

Postoperative Diagnosis: Same

Operation: Open reduction internal fixation distal phalanx left index finger with Kirschner wire stabilization; nonexcisional debridement of laceration of left index finger; repair laceration left middle finger

Procedure: The patient was prepped and draped in the usual manner after an axillary block had been administered. The patient had a Miter saw go into his index finger, lacerating the dorsal radial aspect of the index finger at the distal phalangeal phalanx level. The saw went into the base of the nail. We used the C-arm fluoroscopy to thoroughly evaluate the area and then inflated the tourniquet to 280 mm of Mercury after the arm had been exsanguinated. The wound was thoroughly irrigated with saline solution to which antibiotics had been added and the subcutaneous tissue was debrided of all devitalized tissue, trash, and foreign bodies that were present in the tissue. I then used a Kirschner wire of 0.045 inches in diameter and drilled across the fracture site in the joint to totally stabilize the area. Once this was in place, I then very carefully closed the skin with interrupted running 5-0 Ethibond suture. The area of laceration on the middle finger was just distal to the insertion of the extensor tendon. It looks like the bulk of the nail bed would be viable, but he had some damage to the base of the nail bed. The laceration of the left middle finger, which extended into the subcutaneous tissue, was then repaired with 4-0 Vicryl sutures. A large compression dressing was applied.

(Note: Code only the Medical and Surgical section procedures.)

Code(s): ____

Coding Guideline B4.1a. General Guidelines for Body Part
If a procedure is performed on a portion of a body part that does not have a separate body part value, code the body part value corresponding to the whole body part.

3.41. S01.112 S01.81
Preoperative Diagnosis: Left upper eyelid laceration and chin laceration

Postoperative Diagnosis: Same

Operation: Repair of left upper eyelid and chin lacerations

Procedure: After the patient was suitably prepared under general anesthesia, the left upper eyelid and chin were dressed and draped with Betadine. The left upper eyelid laceration (3 cm) was inspected. It did appear to go through the left upper eyelid canaliculus. The distal end could be seen, the proximal end could not. It was elected not to try to repair the canaliculus. One interrupted 6-0 silk suture was placed through the lid margin and then three interrupted 5-0 Vicryl sutures were placed through the deep tissue. A running 6-0 silk suture was then placed through the skin.

The 2.0 cm chin laceration of the skin was closed with three interrupted 6-0 silk sutures. Gentamicin ointment was applied to the lacerations and a dressing was placed over the left eye. The patient tolerated the procedure well and left the operating room in stable condition.

Code(s): 08QPXZZ 0HQ1XZZ

Coding Guideline B3.1b. General Guidelines for Root Operation
Components of a procedure specified in the root operation definition and explanation are not coded separately. Procedural steps necessary to reach the operative site and close the operative site are also not coded separately.

3.42.
Operation: Transurethral resection of the prostate

Anesthesia: Spinal

Procedure: After operative consent, the patient was brought to the operating room and placed on the table in the supine position. With spinal anesthesia induced, the patient was converted to the dorsolithotomy position. The genital area was prepped and draped in the usual and sterile fashion. A 26 French continuous flow resectoscope sheath was inserted per urethra into the bladder with the obturator in place. The obturator was removed and the resectoscope was seated within its sheath. The bladder was visualized. The ureteral orifices were identified. The resectoscope was pulled to the distal portion of the verumontanum and turned to the 12 o'clock position, and resection of the posterior lobe was begun. Resection of the posterior lobe was carried circumferentially around the glans, channeling a large channel. Hemostasis was obtained by means of electrocoagulation. There were no major venous sinuses or capsular perforations encountered. The verumontanum was left intact. After completion of resection of the posterior lobe, the bladder was evacuated of residual prostatic chips using the Ellik evacuator. The bladder was then visualized. There were no residual chips identified. Ureteral orifices were intact and uninjured. The bladder neck and prostatic fossa were widely patent. Final hemostasis was obtained by means of electrocoagulation, and the resectoscope was removed. A 22 French, 3-way, 30-cc Foley catheter was inserted per urethra into the bladder with ease. It was irrigated until clear. It was placed on light traction with continuous bladder irrigation with sterile water, and the patient was transported to the recovery room in stable condition.

Code(s): ______________________________

Coding Guideline B3.1b. General Guidelines for Root Operation
Components of a procedure specified in the root operation definition and explanation are not coded separately. Procedural steps necessary to reach the operative site and close the operative site are also not coded separately.

Coding Guideline B3.8. Excision vs. Resection
PCS contains specific body parts for anatomical subdivisions of a body part, such as lobes of the lungs or liver and regions of the intestine. Resection of the specific body part is coded whenever all of the body part is cut out or off, rather than coding Excision of a less specific body part.

3.43.
Preoperative Diagnosis: Bronchial alveolar cell carcinoma of the left lung

Postoperative Diagnosis: Same

Operation: Exploratory left thoracotomy; left total pneumonectomy

Procedure: This patient was operated on under general endotracheal anesthesia. We used a double lumen tube where we could selectively ventilate both lungs. He was in the lateral decubitus position. A standard posterior lateral left thoracotomy incision was made and the chest was opened. There was a large diffuse lesion in the left upper lobe periphery. The lesion had previously been biopsied, and we thought we were dealing with a bronchial alveolar cell carcinoma. The man did have a past history of non-Hodgkin's lymphoma years ago, which was presumably cured. I began dissecting on the pulmonary artery to look at things to see what kind of fissure I had developed, but the inner lobar branches were just too dense; that is, there was basically no fissure. I knew if I did a lobectomy, it was really entering the tumor area peripherally. I therefore went ahead and elected to do a left pneumonectomy since his pulmonary function studies were satisfactory preop. The main pulmonary artery was divided between a vascular staple gun. Dissection was a little tenuous. The artery seemed quite friable, but it held nicely. I then reinforced this with a large Chromic tie. We divided the superior and inferior pulmonary vein and prepared for clamping of the bronchus. This completed the pneumonectomy. He tolerated the procedure well. He had some hypotension, but he was hypotensive on induction throughout the entire procedure. Blood gases were satisfactory during clamping of the mainstem bronchus, and he seemed to be reacting well. We closed the chest in layers with Dexon pericostal sutures, approximated clips on the skin.

Code(s): ~~0BTB0ZZ~~ 0BTL0ZZ

3.44.
Preoperative Diagnosis: Localized area of extensive fibrocystic mastitis, upper outer quadrant, right breast

Postoperative Diagnosis: Same

Operation: Partial mastectomy (quadrectomy), upper outer quadrant, right breast

Procedure: The patient was prepped and draped in the usual manner after general anesthesia had been achieved. Local anesthesia with Xylocaine and Marcaine, to which Adrenalin had been added, was infiltrated around the breast to lessen the postoperative pain. This patient had a localized area of extensive fibrocystic mastitis in the upper outer quadrant of the right breast, which was persistently tender. We made an infra-areolar incision around the upper outer quadrant of the right breast and then undermined the skin to the upper outer quadrant. We were able then to carry out a wedge excision of the right breast, removing the full thickness of the breast in a traditional quadrectomy and partial mastectomy type. The specimen was then sent to the laboratory for histological frozen section. This revealed it to be a benign fibrocystic mastitis without any evidence of malignancy. Hemostasis was secured with electrocoagulation, and then the breast parenchyma was secured with electrocoagulation. The breast parenchyma was then reconstructed with 2-0 Dexon suture, followed by 4-0 chromic, and finally 4-0 subcuticular Prolene. A large compression dressing and Jobst mammary support were applied.

Code(s): 0HBT0ZZ

Coding Guideline C2. Procedures Following Delivery or Abortion
Procedures performed following a delivery or abortion for curettage of the endometrium or evacuation of retained products of conception are all coded in the Obstetrics section, to the root operation Extraction and the body part Products of Conception, Retained. Diagnostic or therapeutic dilation and curettage performed during times other than the postpartum or post-abortion period are all coded in the Medical and Surgical section, to the root operation Extraction and the body part Endometrium.

3.45.
Preoperative Diagnosis: Retained placenta

Postoperative Diagnosis: Same

Operation: Manual extraction of placenta

Procedure: The patient was brought to the operating room, where anesthesia was administered. The patient was then placed in the dorsal lithotomy position, prepped and draped in the usual fashion. Exam under anesthesia at this time revealed a dilated cervix and placenta was palpated secondary to previous vaginal delivery. At this time, the placenta was then gently extracted via manual extraction. The placenta appeared to be completely intact.

Code(s): 10D17ZZ

3.46.
Preoperative Diagnosis: Breast cancer

Postoperative Diagnosis: Same

Operation: Port-a-cath placement for chemotherapy infusion

Procedure: The patient was taken to the operating room and placed in the supine position. The right chest and neck were prepped and draped in the usual manner, and 20 cc of 1 percent Lidocaine were injected. The right subclavian vein was punctured, and a wire was passed percutaneously into the superior vena cava. Introducer kit was introduced into the subclavian vein, and the port-a-cath was placed through the introducer and, by fluoroscopy, was placed down to the superior vena cava. Next an incision was made in the chest region over the right pectoralis major muscle superior to the breast and a pocket was created in the subcutaneous tissue. The port-a-cath reservoir was placed into this pocket and tacked down. The catheter was then tunneled through to this reservoir. Hemostasis was achieved, and the subcutaneous tissue was closed with #2-0 Dexon. The skin was closed with #3-0 nylon. The port-a-cath was flushed with saline.
(Note: Do not code fluoroscopy.)

Code(s): ______________________________

Coding Guideline B3.2c. Multiple Procedures
During the same operative episode, multiple procedures are coded if multiple root operations with distinct objectives are performed on the same body part.

Coding Guideline B3.6a. Bypass Procedures
Bypass procedures are coded by identifying the body part bypassed "from" and the body part bypassed "to." The fourth character body part specifies the body part bypassed "from," and the qualifier specifies the body part bypassed "to."

3.47.
Procedure Performed: Subtotal gastrectomy with Billroth II anastomosis

The patient is a 56-year-old male who was admitted with a history of hematemesis for the past 36 hours. He also had some tarry black stools and was noted to have a giant gastric ulcer which was actively bleeding. Patient was subsequently referred for surgical intervention.

Operative Procedure: The patient was brought to the operating room and placed on the table in a supine position, at which time general anesthesia was administered without difficulty. His abdomen was then prepped and draped in the usual sterile fashion. An upper midline incision was made. The peritoneum was then entered using the Metzenbaum scissors and hemostats. A retractor was placed, and he was noted to have a cirrhotic liver with micronodular cirrhosis. The left lobe of the liver was mobilized at that point, and the retractors were placed. On palpation of the stomach along the lesser curvature at approximately the mid portion, there was a large gastric ulcer located just above the pyloric antrum in the body of the stomach. At this point, the gastrocolic omentum was taken off the greater curvature of the stomach to the level of the pylorus. Additionally, the lesser omentum was taken down off the lesser curvature of the stomach to the level of the pylorus. The stomach was then transected approximately 3 cm above the ulcer. At that point, the stomach was reconstructed in a Billroth II fashion by bringing the jejunum through the transverse colon mesentery. Two stay sutures were placed to align the jejunum along the posterior wall of the stomach, and a GIA stapler was used to create the anastomosis without difficulty. The stomach and jejunum were then pulled below the transverse colon mesentery, and this was tacked in several places using 3-0 silk sutures. A feeding jejunostomy tube was then placed distal to this using the feeding jejunostomy kit without difficulty. The abdomen was then irrigated thoroughly using normal saline solution. Hemostasis was achieved using Bovie electrocautery. The midline incision was then closed using #1 PDS in a running fashion. The skin was closed using skin staples. A sterile dressing was applied. The patient was extubated in the operating room and returned to the Intensive Care Unit in guarded condition.

Code(s): 0DB60ZZ 0D160ZA 0DHA0UZ

Coding Guideline B 3.9. Excision for Graft
If an autograft is obtained from a different body part in order to complete the objective of the procedure, a separate procedure is coded.

3.48.
Preoperative Diagnosis: Full thickness burn to right foot

Postoperative Diagnosis: Same

Operation: Split thickness skin graft from right thigh to right foot

Indications: The patient is a 33-year-old male who suffered a full thickness burn to his right foot. The patient has a history of cardiac disease and hypertension. The patient is a 40-pack-a-year smoker who quit 10 years ago. The patient presents for elective debridement of wound and split thickness skin graft.

Operative Description: The patient was taken to the operating room and placed supine on the operating table. After adequate IV sedation was provided, the right lower extremity was prepped and draped in the standard sterile fashion. Sharp debridement of the ulcer was carried out. The ulcer was approximately 4 × 5 cm in area in the lateral dorsum of the right foot. Debridement was carried down to viable tissue. A 4 × 5 cm split thickness skin graft was harvested from the upper aspect of the right thigh. The graft was then meshed and applied to the right foot wound. The graft was secured with a running locked #3-0 chromic suture. Two centrally located chromic sutures were placed for further attention. Attention was placed to the donor site, which was dressed with Xeroform and 4 × 4 gauze. The right lower extremity was then wrapped in Kerlix dressing. Sponge and instrument counts were correct at the end of the case. The patient tolerated the procedure well and was transported to the recovery room.

Code(s): ____________________

Coding Guideline B3.6a. Bypass Procedures
Bypass procedures are coded by identifying the body part bypassed "from" and the body part bypassed "to." The fourth character body part specifies the body part bypassed "from," and the qualifier specifies the body part bypassed "to."

3.49.
Pre- and Postoperative Diagnoses: Arterial insufficiency of the legs

Operation: Aorto-bifemoral bypass graft

Procedure: The patient was prepped and draped, and groin incisions were opened. The common femoral vein and its branches were isolated, and rubber loops were placed around the vessels. At the completion of this, the abdomen was opened and explored. The patient was found to have evidence of radiation changes in the abdominal wall and some of the small bowel. The remainder of the abdominal exploration was unremarkable.

After the abdomen was explored, a Balfour retractor was put in place. The aorta and iliacs were mobilized. Bleeding points were controlled with electrocoagulation. The tapes were placed around the vessel. The vessel was measured, and the aorta was found to be a 12-mm vessel. An 11 × 6 bifurcated microvelour graft was then preclotted with the patient's own blood.

An end-to-end anastomosis was made on the aorta and the graft, using a running suture of 2-0 Prolene. The limbs were taken down through tunnels, and an end-to-side anastomosis was made between the graft and the femoral arteries with running suture of 4-0 Prolene. The inguinal incisions were closed with running sutures of 2-0 Vicryl and steel staples in the skin. The subcutaneous tissue was closed with running suture of 3-0 Vicryl, and the skin was closed with steel staples. A sterile dressing was applied. The patient tolerated the procedure well and returned to the recovery room in adequate condition.

Before the surgical incision was made using the subclavian stick, a Swan-Ganz catheter was percutaneously inserted in the right subclavian vein and guided into the right pulmonary artery. This was sutured in place with 2-0 silk.

Code(s): ______________________________

3.50.
Preoperative Diagnosis: Right trigeminal neuralgia

Postoperative Diagnosis: Same

Operation: Right percutaneous stereotactic radiofrequency destruction of trigeminal nerve

Operative Procedure: After the patient was positioned supine, intravenous sedation was administered. Lateral skull x-ray fluoroscopy was set. The right cheek was infiltrated dermally with Xylocaine, and a small nick in the skin, 2.5 cm lateral to the corner of the mouth, was performed with an 18-gauge needle. The radiofrequency needle with 2 mm exposed tip was then introduced using the known anatomical landmarks and under lateral fluoroscopy guidance into the foramen ovale. Confirmation of the placement of the needle was done by the patient grimacing to pain and by the lateral x-ray. The first treatment, 90 seconds in length, was administered with the tip of the needle 3 mm below the clival line at a temperature of 75 degrees Celsius. The needle was then advanced further to the mid clival line, and another treatment of similar strength and duration was also administered. Finally the third and last treatment was administered with the tip of the needle about 3 cm above the line. The needle was removed. The patient tolerated the procedure well. (Note: Do not code fluoroscopy.)

Code(s): ______________________________

3.51.
Preoperative Diagnosis: Left inguinal hernia

Postoperative Diagnosis: Left inguinal hernia

Operation: Left initial inguinal hernia repair with mesh

Procedure: The patient is a 35-year-old male who presented with several weeks' history of pain in the left groin associated with a bulge. Examination revealed that the left groin did indeed have a bulge and the right groin was normal. We discussed the procedure as well as the choice of anesthesia.

After preoperative evaluation and clearance, the patient was brought into the operating suite and placed in the supine position on the OR table. General anesthesia was induced. The left groin was sterilely prepped and draped and an inguinal incision made. This was carried down through the subcutaneous tissues until the external oblique fascia was reached. This was split in a direction parallel with its fibers, and the medial aspect of the opening included the external ring. The cord structures were encircled and the cremasteric muscle fiber divided. At this point, the floor of the inguinal canal was examined and the patient did appear to have a weakness here. A piece of 3 × 5 mesh was obtained and trimmed to fit. It was placed down in the inguinal canal and tacked to the pubic tubercle. It was then run inferiorly along the pelvic shelving edge until lateral to the internal ring and tacked down superiorly using interrupted sutures of 0 Prolene. A single stitch was placed lateral to the cord to recreate the internal ring. Details of the mesh were tucked underneath the external oblique fascia. The cord and nerve were allowed to drop back into the wound, and the wound was infiltrated with 30 cc. of half percent Marcaine. The external oblique fascia was then closed with a running suture of 0 Vicryl. Subcutaneous tissues were approximated with interrupted sutures of 3-0 Vicryl. The skin was closed with a running subcuticular suture of 4-0 Vicryl. Benzoin and Steri-Strips and a dry sterile dressing were applied. All sponge, needle, and instrument counts were correct at the end of the procedure. The patient tolerated the procedure well and was taken to the recovery room in stable condition.

Code(s): 0YU60JZ

3.52.
Preoperative Diagnosis: Dysfunctional uterine bleeding

Postoperative Diagnosis: Same

Operation: Fractional D&C and Therma-Choice balloon endometrial ablation

Procedure: The patient was taken to the OR and under adequate general anesthesia she was prepped and draped in the dorsolithotomy position for a vaginal procedure. The uterus was sounded to approximately 9-10 cm. Using Pratt cervical dilators, the cervix was dilated to the point that a Sims sharp curette could be inserted. The Sims sharp curette was passed to obtain endometrial curetting. After the curetting was obtained, the Therma-Choice system was assembled and primed. The catheter with the balloon was placed inside the endometrial cavity and slowly filled with fluid until it stabilized at a pressure of approximately 175 to 180 mmHg. The system was then preheated and after preheating to 87 degrees Celsius, eight minutes of therapeutic heat was applied to the lining of the endometrium. The fluid was allowed to drain from the balloon and the system was removed. The procedure was then discontinued. All sponge, instrument, and needle counts were correct. The patient tolerated the procedure well and was taken to the recovery room.

Code(s): 0UDB7ZZ 0U5B7ZZ

3.53.
Preoperative Diagnosis: Right kidney stone

Postoperative Diagnosis: Right kidney stone

Operation: Extracorporeal shock wave lithotripsy of right kidney stone

Procedure: Under IV sedation, the patient was placed in the supine position. The stone in the upper right kidney was positioned at F2. The extracorporeal lithotripsy was started at 19 KV, which subsequently was increased to a maximum of 26 KV at 1,600 shocks. The stone was revisualized, and repositioning was done considering the transverse colon passing right anterior to the stone. Because the stone appeared to be in the same place after the repositioning, shocks were delivered. Apparent adequate fragmentation was obtained after a total of 2,400 shocks had been administered. The patient tolerated the procedure well.

Code(s): ______________________

Coding Guideline B3.11a. Inspection Procedures
Inspection of a body part(s) performed in order to achieve the objective of the procedure is not coded separately.

3.54.
Preoperative Diagnosis: Abdominal pain

Postoperative Diagnosis: Gastritis and duodenitis

Procedure: Esophagogastroduodenoscopy with biopsy

Procedure: The patient was premedicated and brought to the endoscopy suite where his throat was anesthetized with Cetacaine spray. He then was placed in the left lateral position and given 2 mg Versed, IV.

An Olympus gastroscope was advanced into the esophagus, which was well visualized with no significant segmental spasms. Subsequently, the scope was advanced into the distal esophagus which was essentially normal. Then the scope was advanced into the stomach, which showed evidence of erythema and gastritis. The pylorus was intubated and the duodenal bulb visualized. The duodenal bulb showed severe erythema, suggestive of duodenitis. Biopsies of both the duodenum and stomach were obtained. The scope was withdrawn. The patient tolerated the procedure well.

Code(s): ____

3.55.
Preoperative Diagnosis: Cataract, left eye

Postoperative Diagnosis: Cataract, left eye

Operation: Extracapsular cataract extraction with intraocular lens implantation, left eye

Procedure: The patient was given a retrobulbar injection of 2.5 to 3.0 cc of a mixture of equal parts of 2 percent lidocaine with epinephrine and 0.75 percent Marcaine with Wydase. The area above the left eye was infiltrated with an additional 6 to 7 cc of this mixture in a modified Van Lint technique. A self-maintaining pressure device was applied to the eye, and a short time later, the patient was taken to the OR.

The patient was properly positioned on the operating table, and the area around the left eye was prepped and draped in the usual fashion. A self-retaining eyelid speculum was positioned and 4-0 silk suture passed through the tendon of the superior rectus muscle, thereby deviating the eye inferiorly. A 160 degrees fornix-based conjunctival flap was created, followed by a 150 degrees corneoscleral groove with a #64 Beaver blade. Hemostasis was maintained throughout with gentle cautery. A 6-0 silk suture was introduced to cross this groove at the 12 o'clock position and looped out of the operative field. The anterior chamber was then entered superiorly temporally, and after injecting Occucoat, an anterior capsulotomy was performed. The nucleus was easily brought forward into the anterior chamber. The corneoscleral section was opened with scissors to the left and the nucleus delivered with irrigation and gentle lens loop manipulation. Interrupted 10-0 nylon sutures were placed at both the nasal and lateral extent of the incision.

At this point, a modified C-loop posterior chamber lens was removed from its package and irrigated and inspected. It was then positioned into the inferior capsular bag without difficulty and the superior haptic was placed behind the iris at the 12 o'clock location. Then the lens was rotated to a horizontal orientation in an attempt to better enhance capsular fixation. Miochol was then instilled into the anterior chamber. In addition, three or four interrupted 10-0 nylon sutures were used to close the corneal sclera section. The silk sutures were removed, and the conjunctiva advanced back into its normal location and was secured with cautery burns. Approximately 20 to 30 mg of both gentamicin and Kenalog were injected into the inferior cul-de-sac in a subconjunctival and sub-Tenon fashion. After instillation of 2 percent pilocarpine and Maxitrol ophthalmic solution, the eyelid speculum was removed and the eye dressed in a sterile fashion. The patient was released to the recovery room in satisfactory condition.

Code(s): ____

Detailed and/or Complex Cases and Scenarios Using ICD-10-CM and ICD-10-PCS Codes

ICD-10-PCS Coding Guideline B3.13. Release Procedures
In the root operation Release, the body part value coded is the body part being freed and not the tissue being manipulated or cut to free the body part.

3.56.
Preoperative Diagnosis: Carpal tunnel syndrome, left

Postoperative Diagnosis: Carpal tunnel syndrome, left

Operation: Release, left carpal tunnel

Procedure: After successful axillary block was placed, the patient's left arm was prepared and draped in the usual sterile fashion. Tourniquet was inflated. A curvilinear hypothenar incision was made and the palmaris retracted radially. The carpal tunnel and the transverse carpal ligament were then opened and completely freed in the proximal directions. It was noted to be severely tight in the palm with flattening and swelling of the median nerve. The carpal tunnel was opened distally in the hand and noted to be clear. The wound was then closed with 4-0 Dexon in subcuticular tissues. Sterile bulky dressing was applied, and the patient was awakened and taken to the recovery room in satisfactory condition.

ICD-10-CM Code(s): ____________________________

ICD-10-PCS Code(s): ____________________________

ICD-10-CM Coding Guideline I.15.b.5. Outcome of Delivery
A code from category Z37, Outcome of Delivery, should be included on every maternal record when a delivery has occurred. These codes are not to be used on subsequent records or on the newborn record.

ICD-10-PCS Coding Guideline C.1. Products of Conception
Procedures performed on the products of conception are coded to the Obstetrics section. Procedures performed on the pregnant female other than the products of conception are coded to the appropriate root operation in the Medical and Surgical section.

3.57.
This is a 26-year-old patient who had a previous cesarean section for delivery due to fetal distress. During this pregnancy, she has had routine antepartum care with no complications. We are going to attempt a VBAC for this delivery. She is admitted in her 39th week in labor. The fetus is in cephalic position and no rotation is necessary. The labor continues to progress and five hours later she is taken to delivery. During the delivery she is fatigued, so mid forceps are required over a

midline episiotomy which was subsequently repaired by an episiorrhaphy. A single liveborn infant is delivered.

ICD-10-CM Code(s): ___________________________

ICD-10-PCS Code(s): ___________________________

3.58.
Discharge Summary: The patient is a 45-year-old female who fell while walking her dog. She was walking on the sidewalk in her neighborhood and accidently tripped and subsequently fell. She sustained a comminuted fracture of the shaft of her right tibia confirmed by x-ray done in the emergency room. She also hit her head on a fire hydrant and suffered a slight concussion but no loss of consciousness. The patient was admitted and taken to surgery, where an open reduction with internal fixation was accomplished with good alignment of fracture fragments. Postop course was uneventful and the patient was discharged home with daily physical therapy.

ICD-10-CM Code(s):___________________________

ICD-10-PCS Code(s): ___________________________

ICD-10-CM Coding Guideline I.15.b.4. Selection of OB Principal Diagnosis When a Delivery Occurs
When a delivery occurs, the principal diagnosis should correspond to the main circumstances or complication of the delivery. In cases of cesarean delivery, the selection of the principal diagnosis should be the condition established after study that was responsible for the patient's admission. If the patient was admitted with a condition that resulted in the performance of a cesarean procedure that condition should be selected as the principal diagnosis. If the reason for the admission/encounter was unrelated to the condition resulting in the cesarean delivery, the condition related to the reason for the admission/encounter should be selected as the principal diagnosis, even if a cesarean was performed.

Coding Note: Definition of Third Trimester
The third trimester is defined as 28 weeks 0 days of gestation until delivery.

3.59.
Inpatient admission: The patient, gravida II, para 1, was admitted at approximately 33 weeks gestation with mild contractions. She was contracting every 7–8 minutes. An ultrasound showed twins of approximately 4 pounds each. The patient was given magnesium sulfate to stop the contractions, but she contracted through the drug. After developing a fever with suspected chorioamnionitis, a low cervical cesarean section was performed. The umbilical cord was wrapped tightly around the neck of twin 1.

Discharge diagnoses: Cesarean delivery of liveborn twins prematurely at 33 weeks gestation; chorioamnionitis; umbilical cord compression.

ICD-10-CM Code(s): O60.14X0 O30.003 O41.1230 O69.1XX1 237

ICD-10-PCS Code(s): 10D00Z1

ICD-10-CM Coding Guideline II.C. Selection of Principal Diagnosis—Two or More Diagnoses That Equally Meet the Definition of Principal Diagnosis
In the unusual instance when two or more diagnoses equally meet the criteria for principal diagnosis as determined by the admission, diagnostic workup, and/or therapy provided, and the Alphabetic Index, Tabular List, or another coding guideline does not provide sequencing direction, any one of these diagnoses may be sequenced first.

3.60.
This 19-year-old college student was brought to the ER and admitted with high fever, stiff neck, chest pain, cough, and nausea. A diagnostic lumbar puncture was performed, and results were positive for meningitis. Chest x-ray revealed pneumonia. Sputum cultures grew *pneumococcus*. Patient was treated with IV antibiotics and was discharged with the diagnosis of pneumococcal meningitis and pneumococcal pneumonia.

Procedure Note: The patient was placed in the left lateral decubitus position in a semi-fetal position. The area was cleansed and draped in usual sterile fashion. Anesthesia was achieved with 1 percent lidocaine. A 20-guage 3.5 inch spinal needle was placed in the L4-L5 interspace. On the first attempt cerebral spinal fluid was obtained. Four tubes were filled and these were sent for the usual tests. The patient had no immediate complications and tolerated the procedure well.

ICD-10-CM Code(s):________________________________

ICD-10-PCS Code(s):________________________________

3.61. The following documentation is from the health record of a 61-year-old female patient.

Operative Report

Preoperative Diagnoses: Acute gallstone pancreatitis with acute cholecystitis, evidence of bile duct obstruction

Postoperative Diagnoses: Acute cholecystitis with gallstone, acute gallstone pancreatitis, bile duct obstruction

Operation: Cholecystectomy; Exploration of common bile duct; Insertion of feed tube; Intraoperative cholangiogram performed under fluoroscopy

History: The patient is a 61-year-old female admitted 48 hours ago with evidence of possible acute gallstone pancreatitis. The patient had some thickening of her gallbladder wall and pericholecystic fluid. The patient had marked elevation of amylase and was given 48 hours of medical therapy with chemical clearance of her pancreatitis. The patient was felt to be a candidate for open exploration of her biliary tract, with concomitant cholecystectomy and possible common duct exploration.

Description of Procedure: After discussion with the patient and her family and obtaining informed consent, she was taken to the operating room, where, after induction of general anesthesia, the abdomen was prepped and draped in a standard fashion. Following this, a right upper quadrant incision was used to gain access to the abdominal cavity. Manual exploration revealed no abnormalities of the uterus, ovaries, colon, or stomach. The pancreas was enlarged and edematous in the area of the head. Attention was then turned to the right upper quadrant, where the gallbladder was noted to be somewhat distended. This decompressed with a 2-0 Vicryl purse string stitch using the trocar. The cystic artery was dissected free and double clipped proximally, singly distally, and divided. The duct was then dissected free and subsequently clipped proximally.

Low osmolar cholangiogram with fluoroscopy was then obtained by opening the cystic duct and placing a cholangiogram catheter. The common bile duct measured roughly 1½ cm in size. The duct tapered out in the area of the intraduodenal portion of the common duct to near occlusion. The gallbladder was then removed by transecting the cystic duct and removing it in a retrograde fashion. The gallbladder contained several stones.

Following removal of the gallbladder, attention was turned to the common bile duct, which was opened. No stones were retrieved initially from the bile duct. A biliary Fogarty was passed distally and, with some difficulty, was negotiated into the duodenum. On return, no calculus material was obtained. Palpation of the distal duct revealed thickening due to the pancreatic inflammation, which was noted to improve somewhat over the inside portion of the C-loop to the duodenum. The patient was felt to have bile duct obstruction from some other primary duct process other than a stone or inflammation.

Following this, cholangiography revealed some mild emptying of the distal common bile duct into the duodenum. With the overall picture, it was felt the patient might benefit from a feeding jejunostomy, as she might well sustain postoperative or perioperative complications of respiratory insufficiency or perhaps other imponderables. As such, jejunum was identified roughly one foot beyond the ligament of Treitz, and 2-0 Vicryl pursestring stitches times two were placed. The jejunotomy was performed, and a 16 French T-tube was then placed and brought out through a stab wound in the left upper quadrant. The tube was anchored anteriorly with interrupted 2-0 silk stitches and externally with 2-0 stitches. Jackson-Pratt drain was placed through a lateral stab wound in the right upper quadrant and used to drain the duodenotomy and choledochotomy. This was anchored with several 3-0 silk stitches.

Following this, the wound was irrigated with Kantrex irrigation, 1 g per liter, and the wound was closed by closing the posterior rectus sheath with running #1 Vicryl suture. The sub-q was irrigated and the skin was closed with staples. The wound was then dressed, and the patient was taken to the recovery room postop in stable condition. Estimated blood loss was 400 cc. Sponge and needle counts were correct times two.

ICD-10-CM Code(s): ______________________

ICD-10-PCS Code(s): ______________________

3.62. The following documentation is from the health record of a 50-year-old female patient.

Discharge Summary: The patient is a 50-year-old female with known carcinoma of the right breast with widespread pulmonary and bone metastases. She recently completed the third of six outpatient chemotherapy treatments for the metastases. The patient also has a history of a right mastectomy for the breast carcinoma two years ago and is no longer receiving any treatment for this carcinoma. The patient was now admitted for treatment of lumps of the lower-outer quadrant of the left breast. A left mastectomy with bilateral insertion of tissue expanders has been recommended as treatment for the lumps of the left breast due to the patient's history of right breast carcinoma with metastases. The patient has agreed to the recommended treatment.

The patient was taken to surgery, and a left simple mastectomy was performed. Via an open approach, tissue expanders were inserted under both pectoral muscles bilaterally, to start the reconstruction process.

Pathology report revealed benign fibroadenoma.

The patient was discharged in satisfactory condition to see me in the office in 10 days.

ICD-10-CM Code(s): ______________________

ICD-10-PCS Code(s): ______________________

ICD-10-PCS Coding Guideline B3.15. Reposition for Fracture Treatment
Reduction of a displaced fracture is coded to the root operation Reposition and the application of a cast or splint in conjunction with the Reposition procedure is not coded separately. Treatment of a nondisplaced fracture is coded to the procedure performed.

3.63. The following documentation is from the health record of an ORIF patient.

Operative Report

Preoperative Diagnosis: Displaced comminuted fracture of the shaft of the right humerus

Postoperative Diagnosis: Same

Procedure: Open reduction, internal fixation of fracture of shaft of right humerus

History: The patient is a fourth grader whose class was on a field trip at the local bowling alley. The patient tripped over an object on the alley and fell sustaining a fracture of the right humerus.

Description: The patient was anesthetized and prepped with Betadine, sterile drapes were applied, and the pneumatic tourniquet was inflated around the arm. An incision was made in the area of the lateral epicondyle through a Steri-drape, and this was carried through subcutaneous tissue, and the fracture site was easily exposed. Inspection revealed the fragment to be rotated in two planes about 90 degrees. It was possible to manually reduce this quite easily, and the judicious manipulation resulted in an almost anatomic reduction. This was fixed with two pins across the humerus. These pins were cut off below skin level. The wound was closed with some plain catgut subcutaneously and 5-0 nylon in the skin. Dressings were applied to the patient and tourniquet released.

ICD-10-CM Code(s):________________________________

ICD-10-PCS Code(s): ________________________________

ICD-10-PCS Coding Guideline B3.1b. General Guidelines for Root Operation
Components of a procedure specified in the root operation definition and explanation are not coded separately. Procedural steps necessary to reach the operative site and close the operative site are also not coded separately.

3.64. The following documentation is from the health record of a 79-year-old female patient.

Operative Report

Preoperative Diagnosis: Displaced right femoral neck hip fracture

Postoperative Diagnosis: Displaced right femoral neck hip fracture

Operation: Right hip hemiarthroplasty (metal Zimmer LDFX cemented monopolar)

Indications: This is a 79-year-old female that fractured the right femoral neck. The patient was doing some gardening in her back yard when she tripped and fell. The patient lives in a single family home. The patient also has the following chronic conditions: hypertensive heart disease, congestive heart failure, and emphysema.

Procedure: The patient was taken to the operating room and placed in the lateral position on the transfer bed where spinal anesthesia was administered. She was transferred to the left lateral decubitus position on a beanbag on the operative table. Padded all bony prominences. Peritoneum was sealed off with Steri-Drape. The right hip was prepped and draped in the usual sterile fashion. Longitudinal incision over the greater trochanter and proximal femur was performed curving posteriorly proximally along the gluteus maximus. Sharp dissection to the skin, Bovie dissection to the subcutaneous tissues down to tensor fascia lata, identifying the greater trochanter. Besides the tensor fascia lata and along with the incision splitting the fibrous gluteus maximus, controlling bleeders with Bovie cautery. Piriformis was identified and short external rotators were tagged with a #5 Tycron suture. These are moved from their insertion. T-capsulotomy was performed. Displaced hip fracture was identified, femoral head was removed and measured, copious irrigation was performed, and acetabular was visible and palpable, appearing normal. Sagittal saw was used to make cut in the femoral neck. Box osteotome was used to gain lateral entrance to the canal. The canal finder was used, easily locating the femoral canal. Sequential broaching was performed up to a 14, which fit well. Had full range of motion without instability and grossly equal leg lengths. I could bring the hip and knee up to 90 degrees of flexion, neutral adduction, start to internally rotate to 30 degrees before it would become unstable. Hip was redislocated, trial components were removed. I then measured the central canal for a centralizer. I placed a distal cement restrictor 2 cm distal to the component. Copious lavage of the canal was performed and brushed. Acetabulum was irrigated clean, palpable and visibly free of loose fragments. It was packed off with lap sponge. Femoral canal was dried. Cement was placed in the femoral canal with retrograde manner using proximal pressurizer. The 14-mm Zimmer LDFX was placed with a distal centralizer in the appropriate anteversion and held in place with a cement set. Copious irrigation was performed. After the cement set, placed the final endo head, tapped into position with Morris taper, and reduced the head. I could then take the hip through the same range of motion without any instability. The short external rotator is in the drill holes in the greater trochanter. The tensor fascia lata was closed with interrupted 0-0 Vicryl sutures. We copiously irrigated each layer. Subcutaneous tissue was closed with interrupted 2-0 Vicryl sutures, skin was closed with staples. Patient tolerated the procedure well.

ICD-10-CM Code(s): S72.001A, I11.0, I50.9, J43.9
W01.0XXA, Y92.017, Y93.H2 Y99.8

ICD-10-PCS Code(s): 0SRR0JF

3.65. The following documentation is from the health record of an 11-year-old boy.

Preoperative Diagnoses: 1. Ewing sarcoma, left scapula
2. Down syndrome

Postoperative Diagnosis: Same

Procedure: Biopsy of left scapula; Insertion of vascular access device

Findings: This is an 11-year-old boy with Down syndrome who presented four days ago with a large mass in the left scapular region. Outpatient x-ray and CT scan showed laminated new bone with a large expansile permeative lesion in the scapular body. It did not appear to involve the glenohumeral joint. Outpatient bone scan showed marked increased uptake and questionable area of uptake in the right seventh rib and left first vertebral body. At the time of biopsy there was obvious stretching of the posterior trapezius and deltoid musculature over the mass and a very soft calcific mass noted within the central area of the substance. Frozen pathology sections showed many small cells, but definitive diagnosis could not be made off the frozen section. Final pathologic diagnosis was malignant bone tumor consistent with Ewing's sarcoma. He will be started on a chemotherapy program, and definitive surgery will be planned.

Procedure: Following an adequate level of general endotracheal anesthesia, the patient was turned to the right lateral decubitus position with the left side up. The left shoulder region was prepped and draped in routine sterile fashion. Before beginning the biopsy, a vascular access device was inserted into the subcutaneous tissue of the abdominal wall on the right side using an open approach.

A 3 cm incision was then made over the spine of the scapula. Electrocautery was used for hemostasis and the incision deepened with electrocautery. When we were in the area of the soft tissue mass noted on the CT scan, biopsies were taken. The initial biopsies showed primarily muscle fibers, so we deepened the incision at this point and obtained a biopsy of the obvious calcific bone tissue. These cultures were more consistent with tumor, and, at this point, hemostasis was achieved with a combination of bone wax, packing, and electrocautery. Meticulous hemostasis was achieved prior to closure and then a two-layer interrupted closure was performed, closing the skin with a running subcuticular suture of 4-O Vicryl. Bulky dry sterile dressing was applied, and the patient was awakened and returned to the recovery room in good condition.

ICD-10-CM Code(s):____

ICD-10-PCS Code(s): ____

3.66. The following documentation is from the health record of a 32-year-old female patient.

Delivery Record

Admit Note 7/20: Patient is a 32-year-old female with EDC 7/22 and EGA of 39+ weeks. She has been having uterine contractions for 2 days, mild, more severe this a.m. with contractions every 2–4 minutes at admission. Cervix is 1 cm/20%/-1 station. EFW 3,500 g.

Delivery Record Summary 7/21: Patient progressed to 5 cm and exhausted. No sleep for two nights. Patient is also in extreme pain of labor. A vacuum-assisted vaginal delivery of a live male was performed due to the prolonged first stage of labor. A first degree laceration of the perineal skin was repaired with 3-0 Vicryl. Estimated blood loss of 450 ml.

Progress Note 7/22: Patient weak, slightly dizzy, sore perineum. Patient is afebrile and fundus firm. H/H 8.5/24.6. Assessment – s/p VD with first degree laceration; postpartum anemia. Slow Fe #30.

Progress Note 7/23: PPD #2 – S – feeling better, ambulating without dizziness; O VSS, afebrile, fundus firm; A – s/p VD with first degree laceration; P – home today, FU 4 weeks, DC meds Vicodin #20, Colace #20, and Slow Fe #30.

ICD-10-CM Code(s): ____

ICD-10-PCS Code(s): ____

ICD-10-CM Coding Guideline I.C.18.e. Coma Scale
The coma scale codes (R40.2-) can be used in conjunction with traumatic brain injury codes, acute cerebrovascular disease or sequelae of cerebrovascular disease codes. These codes are primarily for use by trauma registries, but they may be used in any setting where this information is collected. The coma scale codes should be sequenced after the diagnosis code(s).

These codes, one from each subcategory, are needed to complete the scale. The 7th character indicates when the scale was recorded. The 7th character should match for all three codes.

At a minimum, report the initial score documented on presentation at your facility. This may be a score from the emergency medicine technician (EMT) or in the emergency department. If desired, a facility may choose to capture multiple Glasgow coma scale score.

3.67. The following documentation is from the health record of a 22-year-old male patient.

Case Summary: The patient is a 22-year-old male, admitted through the Emergency Department after the motorcycle he was driving collided with an elk while driving in the mountains. It was noted that when the accident occurred the patient was driving in the mountains and not on the road. The patient was not wearing a helmet and sustained a skull fracture over the left temporal and orbital roof areas with depressed zygomatic arch on the left side. The patient was unconscious at the scene and upon examination in the ED, with a GCS score of 3: Eyes, never open; No verbal response; No motor response. Left pupil was blown (fixed and dilated), indicating intracranial injury. Hypoxemia, hypotension, and cerebral edema were noted. The patient was admitted to the ICU with continuous monitoring of intracranial pressure (percutaneous). The patient experienced increasing periods of apnea and was placed on a ventilator following endotracheal intubation. The patient's family (in another state) was notified and arrived two days later. There was no improvement in the patient's status over the following five days. The patient continued to be monitored and was unconscious. Attempts to wean from ventilation were unsuccessful. Brain wave measurement showed no brain wave electrical activity. The family made the decision to discontinue life support and the life-sustaining efforts were discontinued.

ICD-10-CM Code(s):____

ICD-10-PCS Code(s): ____

3.68.

This 56-year-old female was admitted for resection of an adrenal mass. The patient has had hypertension of several years' duration. Ultrasound was done on an outpatient basis in consideration of the possibility of a mass, and catecholamine studies have been normal. A 4–5 cm right adrenal mass was identified. Dr. White had obtained a 24-hour urinary free cortisol, ACTH, and short suppression tests, all of which confirmed the presence of Cushing's syndrome. The patient was not diabetic. She did report weight gain, some shift in body configuration, and easy bruising of several years' duration.

Surgery: A 5 cm, well-circumscribed round, benign cortical tumor was resected from the adrenal gland via an open approach. Pathology diagnosis confirmed that the tumor was benign.

Allergies: No known drug allergies

Medications on Discharge: Hydrocortisone, rapidly tapering dose, currently on 40 mg daily; Toprol 50 mg q.a.m.; Prevacid 30 mg qd; Lipitor 10 mg q.a.m.; Prempro 0.625/2.5

Physical Exam: Vital signs stable. HEENT: Sclerae and conjunctivae clear. Neck: Supple. No palpable thyroid. Lungs: Somewhat decreased breath sounds currently. There is mild splinting with deep breathing. Abdomen: Tenderness in the incision area. She has active bowel sounds at this time. Extremities: No definite bruises currently. No edema noted.

Discharge Diagnosis: Right adrenal tumor with Cushing's syndrome secondary to tumor

Plan: The patient appears to have tolerated the surgery well. She will require steroid replacement. Excess cortisol output is presumed entirely due to her tumor, and her ACTH was suppressed previously. As with exogenous steroid therapy, there will be contralateral adrenal suppression. The patient will be tapered rapidly to replacement hydrocortisone levels. We will try the remaining hydrocortisone withdrawal over the next six months or so, depending on her ACTH and cortisol responses. She is discharged to home with follow-up in my office in 1 week.

ICD-10-CM Code(s):____________________________________

ICD-10-PCS Code(s): ___________________________________

3.69. The following documentation is from the health record of a cardiac service patient. Pc only

Discharge Summary

Admit Date: 1/9/xx
Discharge Date: 1/12/xx

Final Diagnoses:	Coronary artery disease (CAD) Sick sinus syndrome Hypertensive heart disease CHF
Procedures:	Percutaneous transluminal coronary angioplasty with stent insertion (1/10/xx) Permanent dual chamber pacemaker insertion (1/9/xx)

History of Present Illness: The patient is a 62-year-old female who was admitted to another hospital on 1/8/xx after experiencing tachycardia. There she underwent a cardiac catheterization, showing the presence of severe two-vessel coronary artery disease. The patient does not have any history of a CABG in the past. The patient has a history of sick sinus syndrome, hypertensive heart disease, and CHF. She was transferred to our hospital to undergo a percutaneous transluminal angioplasty.

Physical Examination: No physical abnormalities were found on the cardiovascular examination. Pulse 50 and blood pressure 100/85. HEENT: PERRLA, faint carotid bruits. Lungs: Clear to percussion and auscultation. Heart: Normal sinus rhythm with a 2.6 systolic ejection murmur. Extremities and abdomen were negative.

Hospital Course: To manage the patient's sick sinus syndrome, a permanent dual chamber pacemaker with atrial and ventricular leads was implanted on 1/9/xx. An incision was made into the left chest wall with the dual chamber pacemaker being placed in the subcutaneous pocket. Next a small incision was made in the skin and the leads were percutaneously passed into the right ventricle and right atrium.

On 1/10 the patient underwent a PTCA of both the left anterior descending artery and the right coronary artery. A drug-eluting stent was placed in the right coronary artery without complications and good results were obtained.

Postoperatively, the patient was stable and was subsequently discharged. The patient's hypertensive heart disease and CHF were managed and monitored during the hospital stay and the patient continued taking her normal medications for these conditions.

ICD-10-CM Code(s): I25. 149.5 I11.0 I50.9

ICD-10-PCS Code(s): 0270342, 02703ZZ (PTCA)
0JH60P2, 02H63MA, 02HK3MA

ICD-10-PCS Coding Guideline B3.2b. Multiple Procedures
During the same operative episode, multiple procedures are coded if the same root operation is repeated at different body sites that are included in the same body part value.

ICD-10-PCS Coding Guideline B3.11a. Inspection Procedures
Inspection of a body part(s) performed in order to achieve the objective of a procedure is not coded separately.

Coding Note: Biopsy Procedures
The qualifier Diagnostic is used to identify excision procedures that are biopsies.

3.70.

Preoperative Diagnosis: Rectal mass
Change in bowel habits

Postoperative Diagnosis: Rectal prolapse
Tubular adenoma of sigmoid colon, biopsies ×2
Sigmoid diverticulosis
Nonspecific colitis

Procedure: Colonoscopy performed to the level of the cecum (110 cm)

Procedure: The patient was prepped in the usual fashion, followed by placement in the left lateral decubitus position. I administered 3 mg of Versed. Monitoring of sedation was assisted by a trained registered nurse. Next, the Pentax Video Endoscope was passed through the rectal verge after a negative digital examination and advanced to the level of the cecum. The scope was then slowly retracted with a circular tip motion. There was mild nonspecific colitis noted. The patient also had significant sigmoid diverticulosis and several small polyps in the sigmoid colon area. Additionally, there was a large prolapsing mass of mucosa approximately 5 cm inside the rectum. This appears to have prolapsed previously. Two of the small polyps were biopsied using the cold biopsy forceps and sent to pathology for examination. The remainder of the exam was unremarkable. The patient tolerated the procedure well.

Pathology Report

Diagnosis: Tubular adenoma of sigmoid colon

ICD-10-CM Code(s): ______________________________

ICD-10-PCS Code(s): ______________________________

ICD-10-PCS Coding Guideline C2. Procedures Following Delivery or Abortion
Procedures performed following a delivery or abortion for curettage of the endometrium or evacuation of retained products of conception are all coded in the Obstetrics section, to the root operation Extraction and the body part Products of Conception, Retained. Diagnostic or therapeutic dilation and curettage performed during times other than the postpartum or post-abortion period are all coded in the Medical and Surgical section, to the root operation Extraction and the body part Endometrium.

3.71.
This 26-year-old gravid 1, para 1, female has been spotting and has been on bed rest. She awoke this morning with severe cramping and bleeding. Her husband brought her to the hospital. After examination, it was determined that she has had an incomplete early spontaneous abortion. She is in the 12th week of her pregnancy. She was taken to surgery, and a dilation and curettage was performed to remove the products of conception. The patient developed a urinary tract infection due to E. coli which was treated with intravenous antibiotics. The patient was subsequently discharged on oral antibiotics and she is to follow up with me in the office.

ICD-10-CM Code(s): ______________________________

ICD-10-PCS Code(s): ______________________________

ICD-10-PCS Coding Guideline B3.6b. Bypass Procedures
Coronary arteries are classified by number of distinct sites treated, rather than number of coronary arteries or anatomic name of coronary artery (for example, left anterior descending). Coronary artery bypass procedures are coded differently than other bypass procedures as described in the previous guideline. Rather than identifying the body part bypassed "from," the body part identifies the number of coronary artery sites bypassed "to," and the qualifier specifies the vessel bypassed "from."

ICD-10-PCS Coding Guideline B3.6c. Bypass Procedures
If multiple coronary artery sites are bypassed, a separate procedure is coded for each coronary artery site that uses a different device and/or qualifier.

3.72.
History: The patient is a 67-year-old male who was transferred from a local community hospital where he was admitted six days ago with chest pain, shortness of breath, elevated cardiac enzymes, and EKG changes indicating an anterolateral ST elevation myocardial infarction. The patient subsequently underwent a cardiac catheterization, which revealed significant four-vessel disease. He was transferred here for a coronary artery bypass procedure.

Past History: Type 2 diabetes (on insulin), hypercholesterolemia and history of carcinoma of the sigmoid colon which was treated with resection of the sigmoid colon and chemotherapy five years ago (the patient has had no recurrence and is currently not being treated). Patient has no past history of a CABG.

Impression and Plan: Anterolateral myocardial infarction, coronary artery disease, diabetes mellitus, and hypercholesterolemia

Operative Report

Preoperative Diagnosis: CAD

Postoperative Diagnosis: CAD

Procedure: CABG ×4; saphenous vein graft to the obtuse marginal, diagonal artery and posterior descending artery; left internal mammary artery to the left anterior descending artery; cardiopulmonary bypass.

Description of Procedure: After obtaining adequate anesthesia, the patient was prepped and draped in the usual fashion. A primary median sternotomy incision was made, and the pericardium was opened. The left internal mammary artery was dissected as a pedicle using electrocautery and small hemoclips at the same time that the greater saphenous vein was harvested endoscopically from the left lower extremity. Cardiopulmonary bypass was instituted and the patient was taken to a mild degree of hypothermia.

The aorta was cross-clamped and electrical arrest effect was administered via cold blood cardioplegia. The saphenous vein graft was placed end-to-side with the posterior descending artery, then a separate graft was placed to the obtuse marginal and finally a separate graft was placed to the diagonal artery. Each anastomosis was done with running 7-0 Prolene suture and verified no bleeders were present. The left internal mammary artery was subsequently brought through a subthalamic tunnel and placed end-to-side with the left anterior descending coronary artery.

Following completion of the grafts, warm blood cardioplegia was administered. During this time, two atrial and ventricular pacing wires were attached to the heart's surface; in addition, mediastinal tubes were also placed. The cross clamps were released following this, and sinus rhythm returned spontaneously. The patient was weaned from cardiopulmonary bypass without incident.

After all grafts were checked for diastolic flow, which revealed no problems, the incisions were closed. The patient was taken to the recovery room in good condition and will be monitored in the intensive care unit. The procedure took approximately 5 hours.

ICD-10-CM Code(s): I25.10, I21.09, E11.9, E78.0, Z79.4, Z90.49

ICD-10-PCS Code(s): 021209W, 0210029, 06BQ4ZZ

LIMA

3.73. The following documentation is from the health record of a 47-year-old female.

Preoperative Diagnosis: Menorrhagia

Postoperative Diagnosis: Menorrhagia

Procedure: Hysteroscopy with biopsy, dilatation and curettage

Indications: The patient is a 47-year-old female with increasing irregular vaginal bleeding. The uterus is very tender, and ultrasound reveals no specific adnexal masses. Pap smear shows some chronic inflammatory cells. Bleeding has not been controlled in the past month with conservation therapy; thus, the patient is admitted for dilatation and curettage, and a hysteroscopy and biopsy will be carried out.

Technique: Under general anesthesia, the patient was prepped and draped in the usual manner with Betadine, with her cervix retracted outward. The vaginal vault appeared to be clear, as did both adnexa. Sound was passed into the intrauterine cavity after the cervix was found to be 8 cm deep. The cervix was dilated with Hegar dilators up to #5. The 5 mm Wolff hysteroscope, with normal saline irrigation, was then inserted. An inspection of the endocervical canal showed no abnormalities.

Upon entering the uterine cavity, some irregular shedding of the endometrium was noted. Endometrial shedding was noted more to be the patient's left cornu area than the right. The contour of the cavity appeared to be normal; no bulging masses or septation was noted. An endometrial biopsy was then taken. The Wolff scope was removed. The cervix was further dilated with Hegar dilators up to #12. A medium-sharp curette was inserted into the uterine cavity and the endometrium was curettage in a clockwise manner, with a moderate amount of what appeared to be irregular proliferative endometrium being obtained. Again, the contour of the cavity appeared to be normal. The patient was transferred to the recovery room in good condition.

Pathology report reveals secretory proliferative endometrium without additional abnormalities noted.

ICD-10-CM Code(s): ______________________________

ICD-10-PCS Code(s): ______________________________

3.74.
Preoperative Diagnosis: Bucket-handle tear left medial meniscus

Postoperative Diagnosis: Bucket-handle tear left medial meniscus

Procedure: Arthroscopic partial medial meniscectomy

Indications: The patient is a 16-year-old male who torn his left medial meniscus while playing football at the local high school football field. The patient is a wide receiver for the high school football team and was tackled resulting in the torn medial meniscus. I saw and treated the patient initially in the emergency room three weeks ago for this injury.

Technique: After induction with general anesthesia, a standard three-portal approach of the knee was evaluated. Mild synovitic changes were noted in the suprapatellar pouch. No chondromalacia changes were noted. The anterior portion of the medial meniscus had a flap tear, which was removed.

After all instruments were withdrawn, 4-0 nylon horizontal mattress stitches were used to close the wound, and pressure dressings were applied. The patient was awakened and taken to the recovery room in good condition.

ICD-10-CM Code(s): ______________________________

ICD-10-PCS Code(s): ______________________________

3.75. The following documentation is from the health record of a 42-year-old male.
Procedure: Left heart catheterization, coronary angiography and left ventriculography

Indications: This is a 42-year-old male who presented to the emergency room with unstable angina and was subsequently admitted. Serial EKGs and cardiac enzymes ruled out a myocardial infarction. The patient has no history of any previous cardiac interventions including angioplasty or CABG. The patient also is being treated for hypertension.

Procedure: The patient was premedicated with 2 mg of Versed in the catheterization laboratory. The right groin was prepped and draped using aseptic technique. The skin and subcutaneous tissues were locally anesthetized with

1 percent Xylocaine. The right femoral artery was entered with 18 gauge needle and 0.035 J guide wire was introduced into the descending aorta. A #6 French left coronary artery catheter was introduced over the guide wire. Selective injections using low osmolar dye were made in the left coronary artery. The right coronary artery catheter was then exchanged with #6 French pigtail catheter and left heart catheterization was performed at rest with pressures being measured. The left ventriculogram was then performed using low osmolar dye. At the end of the procedure, the catheter was removed and pressure held over the right groin until adequate hemostasis was achieved. The patient had good right posterior tibial and dorsalis pedis arterial pulsations following the catheterization. The patient was stabilized and then transferred to his room.

Findings:
Hemodynamics: Pressures: Aortic and left ventricular pressures were normal

Left ventriculography: The overall left ventricular systolic function is mildly reduced. Left ventricular ejection fraction is 40 percent by left ventriculogram. Mild hypokinesis of the anterior wall of the left ventricle. Mitral valve regurgitation is not seen.

Coronary angiography: Left main coronary artery: There were no obstructing lesions in the left main coronary artery. Blood flow appeared to be normal.

Left anterior descending artery: There was a 45 percent stenosis in the mid left anterior descending artery.

Left circumflex: There was a 40 percent stenosis in the left circumflex artery.

Right coronary artery: Right coronary artery is dominant to the posterior circulation. There were no obstructing lesions in the right coronary artery. Blood flow appeared normal.

Impression:
1. Atherosclerotic heart disease with unstable angina
2. Family history of heart disease
3. Tobacco use

ICD-10-CM Code(s): ______________________________

ICD-10-PCS Code(s): ____B215IZZ, B211IZZ____

3.76. The following documentation is from the health record of a 67-year-old male.
Procedure: Placement of a dual chamber implantable pacing cardioverter defibrillator

Diagnoses: Ischemic cardiomyopathy; history of myocardial infarction; status post PTCA

Description of Procedure: After informed consent was obtained, the patient was brought to the cardiac lab. The procedure was done under conscious sedation with fluoroscopic guidance. One percent Lidocaine was used to anesthetize the skin in the left abdominal area and a skin incision was made. A pocket was made in the subcutaneous tissue for the ICD generator, securing good hemostasis. The left subclavian vein was easily cannulated twice using a pediatric set, which was upsized to regular 037 wires, the position which was checked under fluoroscopy.

I then dilated the access volts with 9-French dilators and used 7-French access sheaths through which a 7-French right ventricular lead was advanced and placed under fluoroscopic guidance. It was an active fixation lead. The numbers looked good, and the lead was sutured down.

A 7-French lead was then advanced under fluoroscopic guidance and placed in the right atrial appendage. The numbers looked good. There was no diaphragmatic stimulation and the lead was sutured down. The leads were then attached to the generator, which was tested and sutured down in the pocket. The wound was irrigated several times with antibiotics at the end of the procedure. Wound was closed with layers. The patient tolerated the procedure well without any complications.

The ICD is Model Virtuoso DRD 154AWG. Atrial and ventricular leads are Medtronic. (Note: Do not code the fluoroscopy.)

ICD-10-CM Code(s): ______________________________

ICD-10-PCS Code(s): ______________________________

3.77.
Preoperative Diagnosis: Chronic right calf skin ulcer with necrosis of the bone; E. coli sepsis with acute respiratory failure and disseminated intravascular coagulation (DIC)

Postoperative Diagnosis: Same

Procedure: Right below-the-knee amputation

Description of Procedure: The patient was brought to the operating room and placed supine on the operating room table. The patient was placed under general endotracheal anesthesia. A tourniquet was placed on the right proximal thigh and the right lower extremity was prepped and draped in a standard sterile fashion.

A below-the-knee amputation was carried out directly below the tibial tubercle with a posteriorly based flap. The skin and soft tissue were cut sharply to bone along the line of the skin incision. Once the soft tissue was incised the tibia and fibula were provisionally cut with an oscillating saw and the remainder of the right lower extremity was removed and sent to pathology. Next, the tibia and fibula were dissected out subperiosteally proximal to the anterior portion of the skin incision and re-cut with the oscillating saw. The anterior portion of the tibia was beveled again with the oscillating saw and smoothed with a rasp. The fibular cut was beveled in a lateral to medial direction while extending posteriorly.

The nerves and blood vessels were then addressed. The anterior tibial and posterior tibial arteries, as well as the peroneal artery and attendant veins were suture ligated with #1 Vicryl suture. The anterior and posterior tibial nerves and peroneal nerve were also identified, pulled out of the wound, cut short, and allowed to retract back into the soft tissue. In addition, large veins were identified and ligated. The tourniquet was then released for a total tourniquet time of 32 minutes and minimal bleeding was encountered. Several smaller bleeders were ligated. There was some clotting observed, which was important as the blood clotting was of significant concern preceding this operation. The wound was closed over a medium Hemovac drain with 2 limbs, with the posterior flap brought anteriorly. The fascia was closed using interrupted 1 Vicryl suture, and the subcutaneous tissue was closed using interrupted 3-0 Monocryl suture in a simple buried fashion. Staples were placed at the level of the skin in the interest of time.

After a sterile compressive dressing was placed and Hemovac drain extension and reservoir were attached and activated, the patient was awoken from anesthesia and sent to the ICU in unchanged condition.

ICD-10-CM Code(s): L97.214, A41.51, R65.20, J96.00, D65

ICD-10-PCS Code(s): 0Y6H0Z1

ICD-10-PCS Coding Guideline B3.6a. Bypass Procedures
Bypass procedures are coded by identifying the body part bypassed "from" and the body part bypassed "to." The fourth character body part specifies the body part bypassed from, and the qualifier specifies the body part bypassed to.

ICD-10-PCS Coding Guideline B3.8. Excision vs. Resection
PCS contains specific body parts for anatomical subdivisions of a body part, such as lobes of the lungs or liver and regions of the intestine. Resection of the specific body part is coded whenever all of the body part is cut out or off, rather than coding Excision of a less specific body part.

3.78.
Preoperative Diagnoses: Extensive diverticulitis of sigmoid colon with perforation; Crohn's disease with obstruction of right colon and proximal transverse colon

Postoperative Diagnoses: Same

Procedures: Exploratory laparotomy; sigmoid colectomy; extended right hemicolectomy; colostomy

Procedure Description: After consent was obtained for the procedure, risks and benefits were described at length. The patient was taken to the operating room and placed supine on the operating room table. Preoperatively, the patient received 3 g of IV Unasyn. The patient was placed under general endotracheal anesthesia. PAS stockings were applied to both lower extremities. The patient's abdomen was then prepped and draped in the standard surgical fashion.

A midline laparotomy incision was made from just around the umbilicus to the pubic symphysis. The midline of the fascia was divided, and the abdomen was entered. With exploration of the abdomen, extensive diverticular disease of the distal sigmoid colon was noted.

First order of business was to mobilize the sigmoid colon for a sigmoid colectomy. The left ureter was identified and was far from the area of the sigmoid colon. The sigmoid colon was mobilized laterally to include the area of the diverticulitis. The sigmoid colon was mobilized down to the peritoneal reflection. The medial aspect of the sigmoid colon was also mobilized. The colon was then completely mobilized. A point of transaction was chosen at the proximal sigmoid colon. The mesentery was then taken down across the sacrum. The vessels were tied with 2-0 silk sutures. The sigmoid colon was mobilized down to the proximal rectum. Once the proximal rectum was identified, the sigmoid colon was again transected this time using a contour Ethicon stapler with a blue load. Both the right and left ureters were identified prior to any transection of the sigmoid colon. A 3-0 Prolene suture was then tagged to either edge of the rectal staple line.

The right colon was then inspected. Multiple perforations with sites of deserosalization with exposed mucosa were identified in the right colon. The right colon was mobilized by taking down the white line of Toldt all the way up to and including the hepatic flexure. The omentum was taken off the transverse colon with electrocautery. Once the colon was completely mobilized and became a medial structure, the terminal ileum was transected this time also using a 45-mm GIA stapler with a blue load. A point of transection was chosen in the mid transverse colon just proximal to the middle colic artery where the last site of deserosalization was identified. The mid transverse colon was divided with a GIA 45-mm stapler with a blue load. The mesentery to the right colon and transverse colon were then taken down with Pean clamps and tied with 2-0 silk sutures. The specimen was then passed off the field.

The abdomen was then irrigated. Hemostasis was assured. The ileocolic anastomosis was then created between the terminal ileum and the mid transverse colon. The bowel were positioned to lie along side each other, and a side-to-side functional end-to-end anastomosis was created using a 45-mm GIA stapler with a blue load. The enterostomies were then closed together with a running 3-0 PDS suture followed by interrupted 3-0 GI silks in a Lembert fashion. A stitch was placed at the crotch of each of the bowel connections. A finger was palpated at the anastomosis, and it was widely patent. Mesenteric defect was then closed using 3-0 Vicryl suture in a running fashion.

Attention then turned toward formation of the end-descending colostomy. The descending colon had already been mobilized enough to make it to the anterior abdominal wall without any difficulty. A point on the anterior abdominal wall on the left-hand side just below the umbilicus was chosen for the colostomy. A small 1.5 to 2-cm circular incision was made on the anterior abdominal wall midway through the rectus muscle. The anterior fascia was divided in a cruciate fashion. The rectus muscles were split, and two fingers were palpated through the defect into the abdominal cavity. The descending colon was then grasped with an Allis clamp and passed through the defect and exteriorized. There was no tension on the colon.

On the undersurface of the peritoneum, the colon was tagged with 3-0 GI silk sutures ×2.

The midline fascial incision was then closed with a running #1 looped PDS ×2. The surgical incision was then irrigated with copious saline. The skin was then closed with surgical staples. The ostomy was then matured by removing the staple line and sewing the ostomy in place with 3-0 Vicryl sutures. The sutures were sewn in circumferentially. An ostomy appliance was applied.

Sterile dressings were applied, and the patient was awakened from general anesthesia and transported to the recovery room in stable condition.

ICD-10-CM Code(s): ____________________________________

ICD-10-PCS Code(s): ___________________________________

3.79.

Preoperative Diagnosis: Primary osteoarthritis of right knee

Postoperative Diagnosis: Primary osteoarthritis of right knee

Procedure: Right posterior stabilized total knee arthroplasty

Implants: DePuy Sigma System size 4 right posterior stabilized femoral component, size 3 modular tibial tray with 8 mm. noncrosslinked polyethylene spacer and 35 mm × 8.5 mm thick patella. Antibiotic cement was used.

Procedure Description: After obtaining informed consent, the patient was brought to the operating room whereupon the smooth induction of right femoral block and general anesthesia was performed. The patient was positioned in supine fashion on the operating room table, and all bony prominences were well-padded. A bump was placed under the right hip, and a tourniquet was placed on the right proximal thigh. A gram of Kefzol was given intravenously. The right lower extremity was prepped and draped in standard sterile fashion for arthroplasty including an alcohol pre-prep.

After exsanguinations of the extremity with an Ace wrap, the tourniquet was inflated to 300 mg Hg. An approximately 6-inch longitudinal incision was made about the anterior aspect of the knee centered on the inferior pole of the patella. The skin and subcutaneous tissue were dissected sharply down to the level of the fascia, and a medial parapatellar incision was made in the fascia with the medial most split proximally. The patella was everted, and the knee was flexed. Care was taken to protect the patellar tendon insertion. The osteophytes about the femoral notch were removed and a partial resection of the posterior patellar fat pad was carried out. The femoral canal was entered with a drill, and the sword with distal femoral cutting guide were attached set for a resection of 10 mm. The lateral femoral condyle was noted to be eroded distally and posteriorly; however, a 10 mm cut was sufficient for the distal cut.

Using anterior-referenced system, the femur was sized to a size 4. Rotation was set at 3 degrees external rotation. This was checked using the epicondylar axis. The four-in-one cutting guide was then applied, and the distal femoral anterior and posterior cuts as well as the chamfer cuts were completed. Care was taken to protect the collateral ligaments during these cuts. The femoral notch was then completed using the notch-cutting guide supplied with the system. Once that was done, attention was turned to the tibia. Using an external referenced guide, a tibial cut was made with a zero degree posterior slope with 2 mm off the low (lateral) side. This resection resulted in a similar amount of resection medially and laterally. The tibia was exposed using a Homan placed posteriorly and laterally. The osteophytes were removed laterally and posteriorly.

At this point the osteophytes about the posterior femoral condyles were removed using a curved osteotome under direct visualization. The tibia was then sized to a size 3. A thin cut was then made for the modular tibial tray system. An 8-mm posterior stabilized trial spacer, size 3 tibia tray, and size 4 femur were then applied. The knee was taken through a range of motion. Following this, stability was symmetric medially and laterally. The patella was then prepared. The osteophytes were removed with a rongeur, and the thickness was measured to be 25 mm. An 8.5 mm resection was made down to 16.5 mm and a 16.5 × 35 mm patellar trial was applied after the cut was completed. Stability of this component was then trialed, and it was found to be excellent.

The trial components were removed, and the knee was copiously irrigated with normal saline. The final components were then cemented into place in the sizes mentioned above. Order of cement was patella, tibia, femur. The tibial tray was placed and the knee brought out into full extension to compress the tibial and femoral components. Again, antibiotic gentamicin-containing cement was used. The wound was then cleared of excess cement and bony debris and irrigated one final time. It was then closed in layers over a ConstaVac drain. Number 1 Vicryl was used for the extensor fascia and Scarpa fascia in a simple interrupted fashion, 3-0 Monocryl was used for the subcutaneous tissue in a simple buried fashion, and staples were placed at the level of the skin.

A sterile dressing was placed. The ConstaVac drain extension and reservoir were attached and activated, and a compressive wrap was placed from the toes to the thigh. The tourniquet was released for a total tourniquet time of 112 minutes. EBL was minimal. Postoperatively the patient was taken to the recovery room in stable condition.

ICD-10-CM Code(s): ____

ICD-10-PCS Code(s): ____

ICD-10-PCS Coding Guideline B3.10a. Fusion Procedures of the Spine
The body part coded for a spinal vertebral joint(s) rendered immobile by a spinal fusion procedure is classified by the level of the spine (for example, thoracic). There are distinct body part values for a single vertebral joint and for multiple vertebral joints at each spinal level.

ICD-10-PCS Coding Guideline B3.10c. Fusion Procedures of the Spine
Combinations of devices and materials are often used on a vertebral joint to render the joint immobile. When combinations of devices are used on the same vertebral joint, the device value coded for the procedure is as follows:

- If an interbody fusion device is used to render the joint immobile (alone or containing other material like bone graft), the procedure is coded with the device value Interbody Fusion Device
- If internal fixation is used to render the joint immobile and an interbody fusion device is *not* used, the procedure is coded with the device value Internal Fixation Device
- If bone graft is the *only* device used to render the joint immobile, the procedure is coded with the device value Nonautologous Tissue Substitute or Autologous Tissue Substitute
- If a mixture of autologous and nonautologous bone graft (with or without biological or synthetic extenders or binders) is used to render the joint immobile, code the procedure with the device value Autologous Tissue Substitute

ICD-10-PCS Coding Guideline B3.9. Excision for Graft
If an autograft is obtained from a different body part in order to complete the objective of the procedure, a separate procedure is coded.

3.80.
Preoperative Diagnosis: Degenerative disk disease, L3-4, L4-5

Postoperative Diagnosis: Degenerative disk disease, L3-4, L4-5

Operation: Posterior lumbar interbody fusion, anterior column, L3-4 and L4-5, using BAK threaded fusion cages and Danek pedicle screws with autogenous bone graft

Procedure Description: The patient was brought to the operating room, and after induction of satisfactory general endotracheal anesthesia, he was placed in the prone position on the spinal frame. The back was prepped and draped in the usual sterile fashion.

A #18 gauge needle was used to identify the posterior spinous process of L3-4, L4-5, marked with Indigo Carmine stain and substantiated by x-ray. Just to the left of the midline an incision was made and the incision was carried down through the skin and subcutaneous tissue and fascia. The tissues just under the skin were separated and the left and right lower back muscles were moved aside, exposing the back of the spinal column.

Using the same lumbar incision, dissection of a suprafascial plane was made to identify the posterior superior iliac spine (PSIS). Using an osteotome, the cortical bone of the PSIS was chipped off to expose the cancellous undersurface. A large bone gouge was utilized to harvest the cancellous bone from left iliac crest. The bone is then morselized and stored for use later in the procedure. The graft site was then irrigated with antibiotic irrigation and packed with Gelfoam. The fascial opening was then closed. Laminectomy was then performed.

Next, the fusion was completed using the posterior lumbar interbody technique utilizing BAK instrumentation. The L3-L4 level was addressed first. An alignment guide was placed over the L3-L4 disk space and the disk was incised with a knife. A drill was used to make a hole into the disk space and then spacers were put in sequentially up to a size #11. Cross-table lateral x-rays were then taken of the lumbar spine. A C-ring retractor was placed over the spacer on the left side and the locking tube sleeve was inserted into the body of L3 and L4. The hole was then drilled and loose fragments were moved with the straight pituitary. The BAK was then selected and packed with bone graft obtained earlier from the iliac crest. The bone graft was packed into the cage at the distal end and then the cage was inserted on the left side. The proximal end of the cage was then packed with bone. The same technique was then completed on the right hand side. After completion of the procedure at the L3-L4 level the same technique was done at the L4-L5 level. Because this was a two-level cage procedure, the pedicle screw instrumentation was used to augment the stabilization. The pedicle screw was put into the L3 vertebral body by making a burr hole at the junction of the facet joint and transverse process on the left. The curette was used to make an entry hole into the pedicle and the screw was inserted. The same technique was done on the contralateral side and at the L5 level bilaterally. The screw from L3 to L5 was connected to the other L5 screw with a rod on both sides and then the rods were locked into place with the locking nuts, and the rods were then connected with a transverse connector piece. Final x-rays were taken. The wound was then closed in anatomic layers using interrupted Vicryl suture for the deep layer and staples for the skin. Sterile dressing was applied and the patient was taken to the recovery room in satisfactory condition.

ICD-10-CM Code(s): M51.36

ICD-10-PCS Code(s): 0SG103J 0QB30ZZ

References

American Hospital Association. 1991. *Coding Clinic*, 1st Quarter.

Centers for Medicare and Medicaid Services. 2011a. Development of the ICD-10 Procedure Coding System (ICD-10-PCS). http://www.cms.hhs.gov/ICD10/.

Centers for Medicare and Medicaid Services. 2011b. 2011 *ICD-10-PCS Reference Manual* and Slides. http://www.cms.hhs.gov/ICD10/.

Centers for Medicare and Medicaid Services 2011c. 2011 Official ICD-10-PCS Coding Guidelines. http://www.cms.hhs.gov/ICD10/.

Stedman's. 2006. *Stedman's Electronic Medical Dictionary*. Philadelphia, PA: Lippincott Williams & Wilkins.

Merriam-Webster. 2010. 2006. *Merriam-Webster's Medical Dictionary*. Springfield, MA: Merriam-Webster, Inc.

Dorland. 2007. *Dorland's Illustrated Medical Dictionary*. Philadelphia, PA: W.B. Saunders.

Answer Key

Introduction: ICD-10-PCS Overview

Activity 1: Matching Procedures with Sections

1. Other Procedures
2. Physical Rehabilitation and Diagnostic Audiology
3. Administration
4. Measurement and Monitoring
5. Imaging

Section 1 Review Questions

1. d. 5A2204Z
2. b. False
3. a. Root Operation
4. c. CMS

Activity 2: Identifying Problems with ICD-9-CM Procedure Codes

1. c. Standardized terminology
2. c. Standardized terminology
3. d. Standardized level of specificity
4. b. Diagnosis information excluded
5. a. NOS code options excluded

Activity 3: ICD-10-PCS Key Attribute – Completeness

1.
Character 1: Section is the same for both codes
0 = Medical and Surgical section
Character 2: Body system is different
In 0C9P00Z, C = Mouth and Throat; In 0B0100Z, B = Respiratory System
Character 3: Root operation is the same for both codes
9 = Drainage
Character 4: Body part is different
In 0C9P00Z, P = Tonsils; In 0B9100Z, 1 = Trachea
Character 5: Approach is the same for both codes
0 = Open
Character 6: Device is the same for both codes
0 = Drainage device
Character 7: Qualifier is the same for both codes
Z = No qualifier

2.
Character 1: Sections is the same for both codes
0 = Medical and Surgical section
Character 2: Body system is the same for both codes
B = Respiratory system
Character 3: Root operation is the same for both codes
9 = Drainage
Character 4: Body part is the same for both codes
3 = Right main bronchus
Character 5: Approach is different
In 0B9300Z, 0 = Open; In 0B933ZX, 3 = Percutaneous
Character 6: Device is different
In 0B9300Z, 0 = Drainage device; In 0B933ZX, Z = No device
Character 7: Qualifier is different
In 0B9300Z, Z = No qualifier; In 0B933ZX, X = Diagnostic

3.
Character 1: Section is the same for both codes
0 = Medical and Surgical section
Character 2: Body system is the same for both codes
H – Skin and Breast
Character 3: Root operation is the same for both codes
9 = Drainage
Character 4: Body part is the same for both codes
0 = Skin scalp
Character 5: Approach is the same for both codes
X = External
Character 6: Device is different
In 0H90X0Z, 0 = Drainage device; In 0H90XZZ, Z = No device
Character 7: Qualifier is the same for both codes
Z = No qualifier

Activity 4: Approach Definitions

1. Percutaneous
2. Via Natural or Artificial Opening with Percutaneous Endoscopic Assistance
3. Percutaneous Endoscopic
4. Via Natural or Artificial Opening Endoscopic
5. Via Natural or Artificial Opening

Section 2 Review Questions

1. a. Multiaxial structure

2. a. True

3. d. Limited NEC code options

Activity 5: Root Operations

1. Detachment
2. Excision
3. Removal
4. Revision
5. Extraction

Activity 6: Medical and Surgical Approaches

1. Method
2. Skin
3. 3
4. 7

Activity 7: Coding Exercise

1. 0DB68ZX
2. 0FT44ZZ
3. 0HBU0ZZ
4. 041L0KL

Section 3 Review Questions

1. c. Musculoskeletal System
2. a. Removal
3. b. False

Activity 8: Coding Exercise

1. 3E1U38Z
   Index Irrigation, Joint, Irrigation Substance (3E1U38Z)
2. 10T24ZZ
   Index Resection, Products of conception, ectopic (10T2)
3. 3E1M39Z
   Index: Dialysis, Peritoneal (3E1M39Z)
4. 5A1945Z
   Index: Mechanical ventilation, *see* Performance, Respiratory 5A19
   Performance, Respiratory, 24-96 Consecutive Hours, Ventilation 5A1945Z

Activity 9: Root Operations in the Medical and Surgical-related Sections

1. Dressing
2. Measurement
3. Performance
4. Hypothermia
5. Irrigation

Section 4 Review Questions

1. b. Holter monitoring
2. a. Function
3. a. True

Section 5 Review Questions

1. c. Routine fetal ultrasound, second trimester, twin gestation
2. d. Isotope
3. a. True

Activity 10: ICD-10-PCS Coding Guidelines

1. e. Multiple procedures
2. e. Multiple procedures
3. d. Excision vs. Resection
4. b. Approach
5. c. Device

Section 6 Review Questions

1. b. False
2. b. Guideline B3.11a Inspection of a body part(s) performed in order to achieve the objective of a procedure is not coded separately
3. b. The site, left hand

Final Review Questions

1. c. Single axis
2. d. Seven characters long
3. b. False
4. b. Characters
5. b. Section value D
6. d. Four columns and a varying number of rows
7. a. True
8. b. 10E0XZZ
9. a. True
10. a. True
11. b. Standardized terminology
12. a. Total mastectomy
13. c. Entry, by puncture or minor incision, of instrumentation through the skin or mucous membrane and/or any other body layers necessary to reach and visualize the site of the procedure.
14. c. Diagnostic
15. b. Revision
16. b. False
17. d. Epidural injection of mixed steroid and local anesthetic for pain control
18. a. True
19. d. Obstetrics
20. a. True

Part I: ICD-10-PCS Coding

ICD-10-PCS Training – Day 1

ICD-10-PCS Guidelines and Root Operations Review

ICD-10-PCS Guidelines

1. a. True
2. b. False
3. b. False
4. b. False
5. a. True
6. b. False
7. a. True
8. b. False
9. a. True
10. a. True

Root Operations

11. a. True
12. a. True
13. a. True
14. b. False
15. a. True
16. b. False
17. a. True
18. a. True
19. a. True
20. b. False

Coding Procedures in the Medical and Surgical Section – Section 0

2.1.	0HBCXZZ	Root Operation: Excision Excision, Skin, Upper Arm, Left (0HBCXZ)
	0HBFXZZ	Root Operation: Excision Excision, Skin, Hand, Right (0HBFXZ)
2.2.	0TB43ZX	Root Operation: Excision Excision, Kidney Pelvis, Left (0TB4)
2.3.	0DBN8ZZ	Root Operation: Excision Excision, Colon, Sigmoid (0DBN)
2.4.	0DTM0ZZ	Root Operation: Resection Resection, Colon, Descending (0DTM)
2.5.	0HTT0ZZ	Root Operation: Resection Resection, Breast, Right (0HTT0ZZ)
	0HBT3ZX	Root Operation: Excision Excision, Breast, Right (0HBT)
2.6.	0FT40ZZ	Root Operation: Resection Resection, Gallbladder (0FT4)
	0FJ44ZZ	Root Operation: Inspection Inspection, Gallbladder (0FJ4)
2.7.	07T50ZZ	Root Operation: Resection Resection, Lymphatic, Axillary, Right (07T5)
2.8.	0X6C0ZZ	Root Operation: Detachment Detachment, Elbow Region, Left (0X6C0ZZ)
2.9.	0Y6M0Z0	Root Operation: Detachment Detachment, Foot, Right (0Y6M0Z)
2.10.	0Y6M0Z9	Root Operation: Detachment Detachment, Foot, Right (0Y6M0Z)
2.11.	0U5B4ZZ	Root Operation: Destruction Destruction, Endometrium (0U5B)
	0U574ZZ	Root Operation: Destruction Destruction, Fallopian Tubes, Bilateral (0U57)
2.12.	02583ZZ	Root Operation: Destruction Destruction, Conduction Mechanism (0258)
2.13.	0H5GXZD	Root Operation: Destruction Destruction, Skin, Hand, Left (0H5GXZ)
	0H5FXZZ	Root Operation: Destruction Destruction, Skin, Hand, Right (0H5FXZ)

2.14.	0HD6XZZ	Root Operation: Extraction Extraction, Skin, Back (0HD6XZZ)
2.15.	0CDXXZ2	Root Operation: Extraction Extraction, Tooth, Lower (0CDXXZ)
	0CDWXZ2	Root Operation: Extraction Extraction, Tooth, Upper (0CDWXZ)
2.16.	0JDL3ZZ	Root Operation: Extraction Extraction, Subcutaneous Tissue and Fascia, Upper Leg, Right (0JDL)
2.17.	0D9QXZZ	Root Operation: Drainage Drainage, Anus (0D9Q)
2.18.	0S9900Z	Root Operation: Drainage Drainage, Joint, Hip, Right (0S99)
2.19.	0W9G3ZX	Root Operation: Drainage Drainage, Peritoneal Cavity (0W9G)
2.20.	03C93ZZ	Root Operation: Extirpation Extirpation, Artery, Ulnar, Right (03C9)
2.21.	09CKXZZ	Root Operation: Extirpation Extirpation, Nose (09CK)
2.22.	0HCFXZZ	Root Operation: Extirpation Extirpation, Skin, Hand, Right (0HCFXZZ)
2.23.	0TF7XZZ	Root Operation: Fragmentation Fragmentation, Ureter, Left (0TF7)
	0TF6XZZ	Root Operation: Fragmentation Fragmentation, Ureter, Right (0TF6)
2.24.	0TFC8ZZ	Root Operation: Fragmentation Fragmentation, Bladder Neck (0TFC)
2.25.	0FF98ZZ	Root Operation: Fragmentation Fragmentation, Duct, Common Bile (0FF9)
2.26.	0P8M0ZZ	Root Operation: Division Division, Carpal, Right (0P8M)
	0P8M0ZZ	Root Operation: Division Division, Carpal, Right (0P8M)
2.27.	0L8P3ZZ	Root Operation: Division Division, Tendon, Lower Leg, Left (0L8P)
2.28.	0MN14ZZ	Root Operation: Release Release, Bursa and Ligament, Shoulder, Right (0MN1)

2.29.	0UN24ZZ	Root Operation: Release Release, Ovaries, Bilateral (0UN2)
	0UN74ZZ	Root Operation: Release Release, Fallopian Tubes, Bilateral (0UN7)
2.30.	01N50ZZ	Root Operation: Release Release, Nerve, Median (01N5)
2.31.	0FY00Z0	Root Operation: Transplantation Transplantation, Liver (0FY00Z)
2.32.	0BYM0Z0	Root Operation: Transplantation Transplantation, Lung, Bilateral (0BYM0Z)
2.33.	09M1XZZ	Root Operation: Reattachment Reattachment, Ear, Left (09M1XZZ)
2.34.	0XMJ0ZZ	Root Operation: Reattachment Reattachment, Hand, Right (0XMJ0ZZ)
2.35.	0LXW0ZZ	Root Operation: Transfer Transfer, Tendon, Foot, Left (0LXW)
2.36.	01X64Z5	Root Operation: Transfer Transfer, Nerve, Radial (01X6)
2.37.	0HX5XZZ	Root Operation: Transfer Transfer, Skin, Chest (0HX5XZZ)
2.38.	0VSC3ZZ	Root Operation: Reposition Reposition, Testis, Bilateral (0VSC)
2.39.	0PSC0ZZ	Root Operation: Reposition Reposition, Humeral Head, Right (0PSC)
2.40.	0MSN4ZZ	Root Operation: Reposition Reposition, Bursa and Ligament, Knee, Right (0MSN)
2.41.	0QS734Z	Root Operation: Reposition Reposition, Femur, Upper, Left (0QS7)
2.42.	0UVC7ZZ	Root Operation: Restriction Restriction, Cervix (0UVC)
2.43.	03VG0CZ	Root Operation: Restriction Restriction, Artery, Intracranial (03VG)
2.44.	0UL74CZ	Root Operation: Occlusion Occlusion, Fallopian Tubes, Bilateral (0UL7)
2.45.	05LQ3ZZ	Root Operation: Occlusion Occlusion, Vein, External Jugular, Left (05LQ)

2.46. 03L70ZZ Root Operation: Occlusion
Occlusion, Artery, Brachial Artery, Right (03L7)

2.47. 0F798ZZ Root Operation: Dilation
Dilation, Duct, Common Bile (0F79)

2.48. 037B3ZZ Root Operation: Dilation
Dilation, Artery, Radial, Right (037B)

2.49. 0C7S8ZZ Root Operation: Dilation
Dilation, Larynx (0C7S)

2.50. 02703DZ
02703ZZ Root Operation: Dilation
Dilation, Artery, Coronary, One Site (0270)

2.51. 0D160ZA Root Operation: Bypass
Bypass, Stomach (0D16)

2.52. 041K0KN Root Operation: Bypass
Bypass, Artery, Femoral, Right (041K)

2.53. 0T170ZC Root Operation: Bypass
Bypass, Ureter, Left (0T17)
0T570ZZ Root Operation: Destruction
Destruction, Ureter, Left (0T57)

2.54. 02100Z9 Root Operation: Bypass
Bypass, Artery, Coronary, One Site (0210)

2.55. 021209W Root Operation: Bypass
Bypass, Artery, Coronary, Three Sites (0212)
06BQ4ZZ Root Operation: Excision
Excision, Vein, Greater Saphenous, Left (06BQ)

2.56. 0D1M0Z4 Root Operation: Bypass
Bypass, Colon, Descending (0D1M)

2.57. 0JH60P1 Root Operation: Insertion
Insertion of device in, Subcutaneous Tissue and Fascia, Chest, Pacemaker, Single Chamber Rate Responsive (0JH6)

2.58. 0QHY3MZ Root Operation: Insertion
Insertion of device in, Bone, Lower (0QHY)

2.59. 02H73MA Root Operation: Insertion
Insertion of device in, Atrium, Left (02H7)

2.60. 0SRD0JZ Root Operation: Replacement
Replacement, Joint, Knee, Left (0SRD0)

2.61.	08R93KZ	Root Operation: Replacement Replacement, Cornea, Left (08R9)
2.62.	0HRT076	Root Operation: Replacement Replacement, Breast, Right (0HRT)
2.63.	02RF08Z	Root Operation: Replacement Replacement, Valve, Aortic (02RF)
2.64.	0YU54JZ	Root Operation: Supplement Supplement, Inguinal Region, Right (0YU5)
2.65.	0UUG0JZ	Root Operation: Supplement Supplement, Vagina (0UUG)
2.66.	0SUR09Z	Root Operation: Supplement Supplement, Joint, Hip, Right, Femoral Surface (0SUR)
	0SP909Z	Root Operation: Removal Removal of device from, Joint, Hip, Right (0SP9)
2.67.	0B21XFZ	Root Operation: Change Change device in, Trachea (0B21)
2.68.	0W29X0Z	Root Operation: Change Change device in, Cavity, Pleural, Right (0W29X)
2.69.	0T2BX0Z	Root Operation: Change Change device in, Bladder (0T2BX)
2.70.	0BP1XEZ	Root Operation: Removal Removal of device from, Trachea (0BP1)
2.71.	0PPDX5Z	Root Operation: Removal Removal of device from, Humeral Head, Left (0PPD)
2.72.	0DP6XUZ	Root Operation: Removal Removal of device from, Stomach (0DP6)
2.73.	0TP98DZ	Root Operation: Removal Removal of device from, Ureter (0TP9)
2.74.	0SWB0JZ	Root Operation: Revision Revision of device in, Joint, Hip, Left (0SWB)
2.75.	02WA3MZ	Root Operation: Revision Revision of device in, Heart (02WA)
2.76.	0BJ08ZZ	Root Operation: Inspection Inspection, Tracheobronchial Tree (0BJ0)
2.77.	0DJD7ZZ	Root Operation: Inspection Inspection, Intestinal Tract, Lower (0DJD)

2.78. 0FJ00ZZ Root Operation: Inspection
Inspection, Liver (0FJ0)

2.79. 0DJD8ZZ Root Operation: Inspection
Inspection, Intestinal Tract, Lower (0DJD)

2.80. 0TJ98ZZ Root Operation: Inspection
Inspection, Ureter (0TJ9)

2.81. 02K83ZZ Root Operation: Map
Map, Conduction Mechanism (02K8)

2.82. 00K00ZZ Root Operation: Map
Map, Brain (00K0)

2.83. 0X380ZZ Root Operation: Control
Control postprocedural bleeding in, Arm, Upper, Right (0X38)

2.84. 0W3H0ZZ Root Operation: Control
Control postprocedural bleeding in, Retroperitoneum (0W3H)

2.85. 0HQ3XZZ Root Operation: Repair
Repair, Skin, Ear, Left (0HQ3XZZ)

2.86. 0WQ80ZZ Root Operation: Repair
Repair, Chest Wall (0WQ8)

2.87. 01Q50ZZ Root Operation: Repair
Repair, Nerve, Median (01Q5)

2.88. ~~0SG1031~~ 0SG103J Root Operation: Fusion
Fusion, Lumbar Vertebral, 2 or more (0SG1)

2.89. 0SGP34Z Root Operation: Fusion
Fusion, Toe Phalangeal, Right (0SGP)

2.90. 0W0F0ZZ Root Operation: Alteration
Alteration, Abdominal Wall (0W0F)

2.91. 0H0V0JZ Root Operation: Alteration
Alteration, Breast, Bilateral (0H0V)

2.92. 0J0L3ZZ Root Operation: Alteration
Alteration, Subcutaneous Tissue and Fascia, Upper Leg, Right (0J0L)
0J0M3ZZ Root Operation: Alteration
Alteration, Subcutaneous Tissue and Fascia, Upper Leg, Left (0J0M)

2.93. 0W4N0K1 Root Operation: Creation
Creation, Female (0W4N0)

2.94. 0W4M0J0 Root Operation: Creation
Creation, Male (0W4M0)

Part II: ICD-10-PCS Coding

ICD-10-PCS Training – Day 2

Procedures in the Medical and Surgical-related Sections

Coding Procedures in the Obstetrics Section – Section 1

3.1. 10A07Z6 Root Operation: Abortion
Abortion, Vacuum (10A07Z6)

3.2. 10E0XZZ Root Operation: Delivery
Delivery, Manually assisted (10E0XZZ)

3.3. 10903ZA Drainage, Products of Conception, Fetal Cerebrospinal Fluid (1090)

Coding Procedures in the Placement Section – Section 2

3.4. 2Y41X5Z Root Operation: Packing
Packing, Nasal (2Y41X5Z)

3.5. 2W3FX1Z Root Operation: Immobilization
Immobilization, Hand, Left (2W3FX)

3.6. 2W1RX7Z Root Operation: Compression
Compression, Leg, Lower, Left (2W1RX)

3.7. 2W24X4Z Root Operation: Dressing
Dressing, Chest Wall (2W24X4Z)

3.8. 2W6LX0Z Root Operation: Traction
Traction, Extremity, Lower, Right (2W6LX)

Coding Procedures in the Administration Section – Section 3

3.9. 30243G1 Root Operation: Transfusion
Transfusion, Vein, Central, Bone Marrow (3024)
Bone Marrow Transplant, *see* Transfusion

3.10. 30243N0 Root Operation: Transfusion
Transfusion, Vein, Central, Blood, Red Cells (3024)

3.11. 3E1M39Z Root Operation: Irrigation
Irrigation, Peritoneal Cavity, Dialysate (3E1M39Z)
Dialysis, Peritoneal (3E1M39Z)

3.12. 3E1U38Z Root Operation: Irrigation
Irrigation, Joint, Irrigating Substance (3E1U38Z)

3.13. 3E0S33Z Root Operation: Introduction
Introduction, Epidural Space, Anti-inflammatory (3E0S33Z)
Injection, *see* Introduction

Coding Procedures in the Measurement and Monitoring Section – Section 4

3.14. 4A023N7 Measurement, Cardiac, Sampling and Pressure, Left Heart (4A02)
Catheterization, Heart *see* Measurement, Cardiac (4A02)

3.15. 4A12X45 Root Operation: Monitoring
Monitoring, Cardiac, Electrical Activity, Ambulatory (4A12X45)
Holter Monitoring (4A12X45)

3.16. 4A1H7CZ Root Operation: Monitoring
Monitoring, Products of Conception, Cardiac, Rate (4A1H)

Coding Procedures in the Extracorporeal Assistance and Performance Section – Section 5

3.17. 5A02210 Root Operation: Assistance
Assistance, Cardiac, Continuous, Balloon Pump (5A02210)
IABP (Intra-aortic balloon pump), *see* Assistance, Cardiac (5A02)

3.18. 5A1D00Z Root Operation: Performance
Performance, Urinary, Single, Filtration (5A1D00Z)
Hemodialysis (5A1D00Z)
Dialysis, Hemodialysis (5A1D00Z)

3.19. 5A1221Z Root Operation: Performance
Performance, Cardiac, Continuous, Output (5A1221Z)
5A1935Z Root Operation: Performance
Performance, Respiratory, Less than 24 Consecutive Hours, Ventilation (5A1935Z)

3.20. 5A2204Z Root Operation: Restoration
Restoration, Cardiac, Single, Rhythm (5A2204Z)
Cardioversion (5A2204Z)

Coding Procedures in the Extracorporeal Therapies Section – Section 6

3.21. 6A4Z0ZZ Root Operation: Hypothermia
Hypothermia, Whole Body (6A4Z)

3.22. 6A800ZZ Root Operation: Ultraviolet Light Therapy
Ultraviolet Light Therapy, Skin (6A80)

Coding Procedures in the Osteopathic Section – Section 7

3.23. 7W04X4Z Root Operation: Osteopathic Treatment
Osteopathic Treatment, Sacrum (7W04X)

Coding Procedures in the Other Procedures Section – Section 8

3.24. 8E0W8CZ Root Operation: Other Procedures
Robotic-Assisted Procedure, Trunk Region (8E0W)

3.25. 8E0YXY8 Root Operation: Other Procedures
Suture Removal, Extremity, Lower (8E0YXY8)

Coding Procedures in the Chiropractic Section – Section 9

3.26. 9WB3XJZ Root Operation: Manipulation
Manipulation, Chiropractic, *use* Chiropractic Manipulation
Chiropractic Manipulation, Lumbar (9WB3X)

Procedures in the Ancillary Sections

Coding Procedures in the Imaging Section – Section B

3.27. BG34Y0Z Root Operation: Magnetic Resonance Imaging (MRI)
Magnetic Resonance Imaging (MRI), Gland, Thyroid (BG34)

3.28. BW03ZZZ Root Operation: Plain Radiography
Plain Radiography, Chest (BW03ZZZ)
X-ray, *use* Plain Radiography
Radiography, *use* Plain Radiography
Imaging, diagnostic, *use* Plain Radiography

Coding Procedures in the Nuclear Medicine Section – Section C

3.29. C23GKZZ Root Operation: Positron Emission Tomographic (PET) Imaging
Positron Emission Tomographic (PET) Imaging, Myocardium (C23G)
PET Scan, *use* Positron Emission Tomographic (PET) Imaging

3.30. C7221ZZ Root Operation: Tomographic (Tomo) Nuclear Medicine Imaging
Tomographic (Tomo) Nuclear Medicine Imaging, Spleen (C722)

Coding Procedures in the Radiation Oncology Section – Section D

3.31. DV1097Z — Root Operation: Brachytherapy
Brachytherapy, Prostate (DV10)

3.32. DDY07ZZ — Root Operation: Contact Radiation
Contact Radiation, Esophagus (DDY07ZZ)

Coding Procedures in the Physical Rehabilitation and Diagnostic Audiology Section – Section F

3.33. F08L5BZ — Root Operation: Activities of Daily Living Treatment
Activities of Daily Living Treatment (F08)

3.34. F13Z31Z — Root Operation: Hearing Assessment
Hearing Assessment (F13Z)
Assessment, Hearing, *see* Hearing Assessment, Diagnostic Audiology (F13)
Audiometry, *see* Hearing Assessment, Diagnostic Audiology (F13)

Coding Procedures in the Mental Health Section – Section G

3.35. GZB3ZZZ — Root Operation: Electroconvulsive Therapy
Electroconvulsive Therapy, Bilateral-Multiple Seizures (GZB3ZZZ)

3.36. GZ11ZZZ — Root Operation: Psychological Tests
Psychological Tests, Personality and Behavioral (GZ11ZZZ)
Testing, Mental health, *use* Psychological Tests

Coding Procedures in the Substance Abuse Treatment Section – Section H

3.37. HZ2ZZZZ — Root Operation: Detoxification Services
Detoxification Services, for substance abuse (HZ2ZZZZ)

3.38. HZ53ZZZ — Root Operation: Psychotherapy
Psychotherapy, Individual, for substance abuse, 12-Step (HZ53ZZZ)

Case Studies from Inpatient Health Records

3.39. 0UT90ZZ — Resection, Uterus (0UT9)
Hysterectomy, *see* Resection, Uterus (0UT9)
0UTC0ZZ — Resection, Cervix (0UTC)
0UT20ZZ — Resection, Ovary, Bilateral (0UT2)
0UT70ZZ — Resection, Fallopian Tubes, Bilateral (0UT7)
0FB20ZX — Excision, Liver, Left Lobe (0FB2)
Biopsy, *see* Excision, diagnostic

3.40.	0PSV04Z	Reposition, Phalanx, Finger, Left (0PSV) Reduction, Fracture, *see* Reposition
	0JDK0ZZ	Extraction, Subcutaneous Tissue and Fascia, Hand, Left (0JDK) Debridement, Non-Excisional, *see* Extraction
	0JQK0ZZ	Repair, Subcutaneous Tissue and Fascia, Hand, Left (0JQK) Suture, Laceration repair, *see* Repair
3.41.	08QPXZZ	Repair, Eyelid, Upper, Left (08QP) Suture, Laceration repair, *see* Repair
	0HQ1XZZ	Repair, Skin, Face (0HQ1XZZ)
3.42.	0VB08ZZ	Excision, Prostate (0VB0) Prostatectomy, *see* Excision, Prostate (0VB0)
3.43.	0BTL0ZZ	Resection, Lung, Left (0BTL) Pneumonectomy, *see* Resection, Respiratory System (0BT)
3.44.	0HBT0ZZ	Excision, Breast, Right (0HBT) Mastectomy, *see*, Excision, Skin and Breast (0HB) Quadrant resection of breast, *see* Excision, Skin and Breast (0HB)
3.45.	10D17ZZ	Extraction, by Body Part, Products of Conception, Retained (10D1)
3.46.	02HV33Z	Insertion of device in, Vena Cava, Superior (02HV)
	0JH60WZ	Insertion of device in, Subcutaneous Tissue and Fascia, Chest (0JH6)
3.47.	0DB60ZZ	Excision, Stomach (0DB6) Gastrectomy, *see*, Excision, Stomach (0DB6)
	0D160ZA	Bypass, Stomach (0D16)
	0DHA0UZ	Insertion of device in, Jejunum (0DHA)
3.48.	0HRMX74	Replacement, Skin, Foot, Right (0HRM) Graft, *see* Replacement
	0HBHXZZ	Excision, Skin, Upper Leg, Right (0HBHXZ)
3.49.	04100JK	Bypass, Aorta, Abdominal (0410)
	02HQ32Z	Insertion of device in, Artery, Pulmonary, Right (02HQ)
3.50.	005K3ZZ	Destruction, Nerve, Trigeminal (005K)
3.51.	0YU60JZ	Supplement, Inguinal Region, Left (0YU6) Herniorrhaphy, with synthetic substitute, *see* Supplement Anatomical Regions, Lower Extremities (0YU)
3.52.	0UDB7ZZ	Extraction, Endometrium (0UDB)
	0U5B7ZZ	Destruction, Endometrium (0U5B) Ablation, *see* Destruction

3.53.	0TF3XZZ	Fragmentation, Kidney Pelvis, Right (0TF3) ESWL (extracorporeal shock wave lithotripsy), *see* Fragmentation
3.54.	0DB98ZX 0DB68ZX	Excision, Duodenum (0DB9) Excision, Stomach (0DB6) Biopsy, *see* Excision, Diagnostic
3.55.	08RK3JZ	Replacement, Lens, Left (08RK)

Detailed and/or Complex Cases and Scenarios Using ICD-10-CM and ICD-10-PCS Codes

3.56.	G56.02 01N50ZZ	Syndrome, carpal tunnel Release, Nerve, Median Nerve (01N5)
3.57.	O75.81	Pregnancy, complicated by, fatigue, during labor and delivery
	O34.21	Delivery, vaginal, following previous cesarean delivery
	Z37.0	Outcome of delivery, single, liveborn
	10D07Z4	Extraction, Products of Conception, Mid Forceps (10D07Z4) Delivery, Forceps, *see* Extraction, Products of Conception (10D0)
	0W8NXZZ	Division, Perineum, Female (0W8NXZZ) Episiotomy, *see* Division, Perineum, Female (0W8N)
3.58.	S82.251A	Fracture, traumatic, tibia (shaft), comminuted (displaced)
	S06.0x0A	Concussion (brain) (cerebral) (current)
	W01.198A	Index to External Causes, Fall, due to, slipping, with subsequent striking against object, specified NEC
	Y92.480	Index to External Causes, Place of occurrence, sidewalk
	Y93.K1	Index to External Causes, Activity, walking an animal
	Y99.8	Index to External Causes, Status of external cause, leisure activity
	0QSG04Z	Reposition, Tibia, Right (0QSG) Reduction, Fracture *see* Reposition
3.59.	O60.14x0	Delivery, preterm (*see also* Pregnancy, complicated by, preterm labor) Pregnancy, complicated by, preterm labor, third trimester, with third trimester preterm delivery
	O30.003	Pregnancy, twin – *see* Tabular for required extensions
	O41.1230	Chorioamnionitis; or Pregnancy, complicated by, chorioamnionitis
	O69.1xx1	Compression, umbilical cord, complicating delivery, cord around neck; or Delivery, complicated by, cord, around neck, tightly or with compression
	Z37.2	Outcome of delivery, twins, both liveborn
	10D00Z1	Cesarean Section, *see* Extraction, Products of Conception (10D0) Extraction, Products of Conception, Low Cervical (10D00Z1)

3.60.	G00.1	Meningitis, pneumococcal
	J13	Pneumonia, pneumococcal
	009Y3ZX	Puncture – *see* Drainage Drainage, Spinal Cord, Lumbar (009Y)
3.61.	K80.01	Calculus, calculi, calculous, gallbladder, with, cholecystitis, acute, with, obstruction Cholecystitis, with calculus, stones, in, gallbladder, *see*, Calculus, gallbladder, with cholecystitis
	K85.1	Pancreatitis, acute, gallstone
	0FT40ZZ	Cholecystectomy – *see* Resection, Gallbladder (0FT4)
	0FJB0ZZ	Exploration – *see* Inspection Inspection, Duct, Hepatobiliary (0FJB)
	0DHA0UZ	Insertion of device in, Jejunum (0DHA)
	BF101ZZ	Fluoroscopy, Bile Duct (BF10) Cholangiogram, *see* Fluoroscopy, Hepatobiliary System and Pancreas (BF1)
3.62.	D24.2	Fibroadenoma, specified site NEC – *see* Neoplasm, benign Neoplasm Table, breast, lower-outer quadrant, benign
	C79.51	Neoplasm Table, bone, malignant, secondary
	C78.00	Neoplasm Table, lung, lobe NEC, malignant, secondary
	Z85.3	History, personal (of), malignant neoplasm (of), breast
	Z90.11	Absence, breast(s) (and nipple(s)) (acquired)
	0HTU0ZZ	Mastectomy – *see* Resection, Skin and Breast (0HT) Resection, Breast, Left (0HTU0ZZ)
	0HHV0NZ	Insertion of device in, Breast, Bilateral (0HHV)
3.63.	S42.351A	Fracture, traumatic, humerus, shaft, comminuted (displaced), right
	W01.0xxA	Fall, same level, from, slipping, stumbling, tripping
	Y92.39	Place of occurrence, bowling alley
	Y93.54	Activity, bowling
	Y99.8	Status of External Cause, student activity
	0PSF04Z	Reposition, Humeral Shaft, Right (0PSF)
3.64.	S72.001A	Fracture, traumatic, femur, upper end, neck
	I11.0	Hypertension, hypertensive, heart, with heart failure
	I50.9	Failure, heart, congestive
	J43.9	Emphysema (atrophic) (bullous) (chronic) (interlobular) (lung) (obstructive) (pulmonary) (senile) (vesicular)
	W01.0xxA	Index to External Causes, Fall, same level, from, slipping, stumbling, tripping
	Y92.017	Index to External Causes, Place of occurrence, residence, house, single-family, yard
	Y93.H2	Index to External Causes, Activity, gardening
	Y99.8	Index to External Causes, External cause status, leisure activity
	0SRR0JF	Replacement, Joint, Hip, Right, Femoral Surface (0SRR)

3.65.	C40.02	Sarcoma, Ewing's – *see* Neoplasm, bone, malignant Neoplasm Table, bone, scapula, left side, malignant, primary
	Q90.9	Syndrome, Down
	0PB60ZX	Excision, Scapula, Left (0PB6) Biopsy – *see* Excision
	0JH80XZ	Insertion of device in, Subcutaneous Tissue and Fascia, Abdomen (0JH8)
3.66.	O63.0	Delivery (childbirth) (labor), complicated, by, prolonged labor, first stage
	O70.0	Delivery (childbirth) (labor) (complicated by), complicated, by, laceration (perineal), perineum, first degree
	O75.81	Exhaustion, exhaustive, maternal, complicating delivery
	O90.81	Pregnancy (childbirth) (labor) (puerperium), complicated by (management affected by), anemia (pre-existing), postpartum
	Z37.0	Outcome of delivery, single, liveborn
	10D07Z6	Extraction, Products of Conception, Vacuum (10D07Z6) Delivery, Vacuum assisted, *see* Extraction, Products of Conception (10D0)
	0HQ9XZZ	Repair, Skin, Perineum (0HQ9XZZ)
3.67.	S02.19xA	Fracture, traumatic, skull, temporal bone
	S02.402A	Fracture, traumatic, zygoma
	S06.1x7A	Injury, intracranial, cerebral edema, traumatic
	R40.2312	Coma, with, motor response (none)
	R40.2112	Coma, with, opening of eyes (never)
	R40.2212	Coma, with, verbal response (none)
	V20.0xxA	Index to External Causes; Accident, transport, motorcyclist, driver, collision (with), animal, nontraffic Accident, motorcycle NOS, *see* Accident, transport, motorcyclist
	Y92.828	Index to External Causes; Place of occurrence, mountain
	0BH17EZ	Insertion of device in, Trachea (0BH1) Intubation, Airway, *see* Insertion of device in, Trachea (0BH1)
	5A1955Z	Performance, Respiratory, Greater than 96 Consecutive Hours, Ventilation (5A1955Z)
	4A103BD	Monitoring, Central Nervous, Pressure, Intracranial (4A10)
	4A00X4Z	Measurement, Central Nervous, Electrical Activity (4A00)
3.68.	D35.01	Neoplasm Table: Adrenal, cortex, right side, benign
	E24.8	Cushing's, syndrome or disease, specified NEC
	I10	Hypertension, hypertensive (accelerated) (benign) (essential) (idiopathic) (malignant) (systemic)
	0GB30ZZ	Excision, Gland, Adrenal, Right (0GB3)

3.69.	I25.10	Arteriosclerosis, arteriosclerotic, coronary (artery)
	I49.5	Syndrome, sick, sinus
	I11.0	Hypertension, heart (disease), with heart failure (congestive)
	I50.9	Failure, heart, congestive
	02703ZZ	Dilation, Artery, Coronary, One Site (0270)
	027034Z	Dilation, Artery, Coronary, One Site (0270) Angioplasty, *see* Dilation, Heart and Great Vessels (027) Percutaneous transluminal coronary angioplasty (PTCA), *see* Dilation, Heart and Great Vessels (027)
	0JH60P2	Insertion of device in, Subcutaneous Tissue and Fascia, Chest, Pacemaker, Dual Chamber (0JH6)
	02H63MA	Insertion of device in, Atrium, Right (02H6) Pacemaker Lead, Atrium, Right (02H6)
	02HK3MA	Insertion of device in, Ventricle, Right (02HK) Pacemaker Lead, Ventricle, Right (02HK)
3.70.	D12.5	Adenoma – *see also* Neoplasm, benign, by site Neoplasm Table: intestines, large, colon, sigmoid
	K62.3	Prolapse, prolapsed, rectum (mucosa) (sphincter)
	K57.30	Diverticulosis, large intestine
	K52.9	Colitis (acute) (catarrhal) (chronic) (noninfectious) (hemorrhagic)
	0DBN8ZX	Excision, Colon, Sigmoid (0DBN)
	0DBN8ZX	Excision, Colon, Sigmoid (0DBN) Biopsy, see Excision, Diagnostic
3.71.	O03.38	Abortion (complete) (spontaneous), incomplete (spontaneous), complicated (by) (following), infection, urinary tract
	B96.2	Infection, infected, infective (opportunistic), Escherichia (E.) coli NEC, as cause of disease classified elsewhere
	10D17ZZ	Extraction, Products of Conception, Retained (10D1)
3.72.	I25.10	Arteriosclerosis, arteriosclerotic (diffuse) (obliterans) (of) (senile) (with calcification), coronary (artery), native vessel
	I21.09	Infarct, infarction, myocardium, ST elevation, anterior (anteroapical) (anterolateral) (anteroseptal) (Q wave) (wall)
	E11.9	Diabetes, diabetic (mellitus) (sugar), type 2
	E78.0	Hypercholesterolemia (essential) (familial) (hereditary) (primary) (pure)
	Z92.21	History, personal (of), chemotherapy for neoplastic condition
	Z85.038	History, personal (of), malignant neoplasm, colon NEC
	Z79.4	Long-term (current) drug therapy (use of), insulin
	Z90.49	Absence (of) (organ or part) (complete or partial), intestine (acquired), large
	021209W	Bypass, Artery, Coronary, Three Sites (0212)
	02100Z9	Bypass, Artery, Coronary, One Site (0210)
	5A1221Z	Performance, Cardiac, Continuous, Output (5A1221Z)
	5A1935Z	Performance, Respiratory, Less than 24 Consecutive Hours, Ventilation (5A1935Z)
	06BQ4ZZ	Excision, Vein, Greater Saphenous, Left (06BQ)

3.73. N92.0 Menorrhagia (primary)
0UDB7ZZ Extraction, Endometrium (0UDB)
0UDB8ZX Extraction, Endometrium (0UDB)

3.74. S83.212A Tear, torn (traumatic) meniscus (knee) (current injury), medial, bucket-handle
W03.xxxD Tackle in sports
0SBD4ZZ Excision, Joint, Knee, Left (0SBD)
Meniscectomy, *see* Excision, Lower Joints (0SB)

3.75. I25.110 Arteriosclerosis, arteriosclerotic (diffuse) (obliterans) (of) (senile) (with calcification), coronary (artery), native vessel, with, angina pectoris, unstable
I10 Hypertension, hypertensive (accelerated) (benign) (essential) (idiopathic) (malignant) (systemic)
Z82.49 History, family, disease or disorder (of), cardiovascular NEC
Z72.0 Tobacco, use
Use, tobacco
4A023N7 Measurement, Cardiac, Sampling and Pressure, Left Heart (4A02)
Catheterization, Heart *see* Measurement, Cardiac (4A02)
B2151ZZ Fluoroscopy, Heart, Left (B215)
B2111ZZ Fluoroscopy, Artery, Coronary, Multiple (B211)
Angiography, *see* Fluoroscopy, Heart (B21)

3.76. I25.5 Cardiomyopathy, ischemic
I25.2 History, personal, myocardial infarction (old)
Z98.61 Status, angioplasty, coronary artery
0JH80P4 Insertion of device in, Subcutaneous Tissue and Fascia, Abdomen
Defibrillator Generator (0JH8)
02HK3ME Defibrillator Lead, Ventricle, Right (02HK)
02H63ME Defibrillator Lead, Atrium, Right (02H6)

3.77. L97.214 Ulcer, lower limb, calf, right, with bone necrosis
A41.51 Sepsis, Escherichia coli (E. coli)
R65.20 Sepsis, severe
J96.00 Failure, respiration, respiratory, acute
D65 Defibrination (syndrome)
Coagulation, intravascular (diffuse) (disseminated), *see also* Defibrination syndrome
0Y6H0Z1 Detachment, Leg, Lower, Right (0Y6H0Z)
Amputation, *see* Detachment

3.78.	K57.20	Diverticulitis, intestine, large, with abscess, perforation or peritonitis
	K50.112	Enteritis, regional, large intestine, with, intestinalobstruction Crohn's disease, *see* Enteritis, regional
	0DTN0ZZ	Resection, Colon, Sigmoid (0DTN) Colectomy, *see* Resection, Gastrointestinal System (0DT)
	0DTF0ZZ	Resection, Intestine, Large, Right (0DTF) Hemicolectomy *see* Resection, Gastrointestinal System (0DT)
	0DBL0ZZ	Excision, Colon, Transverse (0DBL)
	0D1M0Z4	Bypass, Colon, Descending (0D1M) Colostomy, *see* Bypass, Gastrointestinal System (0D1)
3.79.	M17.11	Osteoarthritis, primary, knee
	0SRC0JZ	Replacement, Joint, Knee, Right (0SRC0) Arthroplasty, *see* Replacement, Lower Joints (0SR)
3.80.	M51.36	Degeneration, degenerative, intervertebral disc, Lumbar region Disease, disc, degenerative *see* Degeneration, Intervertebral disc
	0SG103J	Fusion, Lumbar Vertebral, 2 or more (0SG1)
	0QB30ZZ	Excision, Bone, Pelvic, Left (0QB3) Iliac Crest *use* Bone, Pelvic, Left

Appendix A

(Note: The Body Part Key by Anatomical Term Table listed in Appendix A contains the same information as presented in Appendix A of the 2011 ICD-10-PCS Reference Manual but is presented in a different format.)

Body Part Key by Anatomical Term

ICD-10 PROCEDURE CODING SYSTEM
MEDICAL/SURGICAL SECTION
BODY PART KEY BY ANATOMICAL TERM

Anatomical Term	PCS Description
Abdominal aortic plexus	Abdominal Sympathetic Nerve
Abdominal esophagus (syn)	Esophagus, Lower
Abductor hallucis muscle	Foot Muscle, Right
Abductor hallucis muscle	Foot Muscle, Left
Abductor hallucis tendon	Foot Tendon, Right
Abductor hallucis tendon	Foot Tendon, Left
Accessory cephalic vein	Cephalic Vein, Right
Accessory cephalic vein	Cephalic Vein, Left
Accessory obturator nerve	Lumbar Plexus
Accessory phrenic nerve	Phrenic Nerve
Accessory spleen	Spleen
Acetabulofemoral joint (syn)	Hip Joint, Left
Acetabulofemoral joint (syn)	Hip Joint, Right
Achilles tendon	Lower Leg Tendon, Right
Achilles tendon	Lower Leg Tendon, Left
Acromioclavicular ligament	Shoulder Bursa and Ligament, Right
Acromioclavicular ligament	Shoulder Bursa and Ligament, Left
Acromion (process)	Scapula, Left
Acromion (process)	Scapula, Right
Acute margin	Ventricle, Right
Adductor brevis muscle	Upper Leg Muscle, Right
Adductor brevis muscle	Upper Leg Muscle, Left
Adductor brevis tendon	Upper Leg Tendon, Right
Adductor brevis tendon	Upper Leg Tendon, Left
Adductor hallucis muscle	Foot Muscle, Right
Adductor hallucis muscle	Foot Muscle, Left
Adductor hallucis tendon	Foot Tendon, Right
Adductor hallucis tendon	Foot Tendon, Left
Adductor longus muscle	Upper Leg Muscle, Right
Adductor longus muscle	Upper Leg Muscle, Left
Adductor longus tendon	Upper Leg Tendon, Right
Adductor longus tendon	Upper Leg Tendon, Left
Adductor magnus muscle	Upper Leg Muscle, Right
Adductor magnus muscle	Upper Leg Muscle, Left
Adductor magnus tendon	Upper Leg Tendon, Right
Adductor magnus tendon	Upper Leg Tendon, Left
Adenohypophysis	Pituitary Gland
Alar ligament of axis	Head and Neck Bursa and Ligament
Alveolar process of mandible	Mandible, Left
Alveolar process of mandible	Mandible, Right
Alveolar process of maxilla	Maxilla, Left
Alveolar process of maxilla	Maxilla, Right

ICD-10 PROCEDURE CODING SYSTEM
MEDICAL/SURGICAL SECTION
BODY PART KEY BY ANATOMICAL TERM

Anatomical Term	PCS Description
Anal orifice (syn)	Anus
Anatomical snuffbox	Lower Arm and Wrist Tendon, Right
Anatomical snuffbox	Lower Arm and Wrist Tendon, Left
Angular artery	Face Artery
Angular vein	Face Vein, Left
Angular vein	Face Vein, Right
Annular ligament	Elbow Bursa and Ligament, Right
Annular ligament	Elbow Bursa and Ligament, Left
Anorectal junction	Rectum
Ansa cervicalis	Cervical Plexus
Antebrachial fascia	Subcutaneous Tissue and Fascia, Right Lower Arm
Antebrachial fascia	Subcutaneous Tissue and Fascia, Left Lower Arm
Anterior (pectoral) lymph node	Lymphatic, Left Axillary
Anterior (pectoral) lymph node	Lymphatic, Right Axillary
Anterior cerebral artery	Intracranial Artery
Anterior cerebral vein	Intracranial Vein
Anterior choroidal artery	Intracranial Artery
Anterior circumflex humeral artery	Axillary Artery, Right
Anterior circumflex humeral artery	Axillary Artery, Left
Anterior communicating artery	Intracranial Artery
Anterior crural nerve (syn)	Femoral Nerve
Anterior cruciate ligament (ACL)	Knee Bursa and Ligament, Right
Anterior cruciate ligament (ACL)	Knee Bursa and Ligament, Left
Anterior facial vein	Face Vein, Left
Anterior facial vein	Face Vein, Right
Anterior intercostal artery	Internal Mammary Artery, Right
Anterior intercostal artery	Internal Mammary Artery, Left
Anterior interosseous nerve	Median Nerve
Anterior lateral malleolar artery	Anterior Tibial Artery, Right
Anterior lateral malleolar artery	Anterior Tibial Artery, Left
Anterior lingual gland	Minor Salivary Gland
Anterior medial malleolar artery	Anterior Tibial Artery, Right
Anterior medial malleolar artery	Anterior Tibial Artery, Left
Anterior spinal artery	Vertebral Artery, Right
Anterior spinal artery	Vertebral Artery, Left
Anterior tibial recurrent artery	Anterior Tibial Artery, Right
Anterior tibial recurrent artery	Anterior Tibial Artery, Left
Anterior ulnar recurrent artery	Ulnar Artery, Right
Anterior ulnar recurrent artery	Ulnar Artery, Left
Anterior vagal trunk	Vagus Nerve

ICD-10 PROCEDURE CODING SYSTEM
MEDICAL/SURGICAL SECTION
BODY PART KEY BY ANATOMICAL TERM

Anatomical Term	PCS Description
Anterior vertebral tendon	Head and Neck Tendon
Anterior vertebral muscle	Neck Muscle, Right
Anterior vertebral muscle	Neck Muscle, Left
Antihelix	External Ear, Right
Antihelix	External Ear, Left
Antihelix	External Ear, Bilateral
Antitragus	External Ear, Right
Antitragus	External Ear, Left
Antitragus	External Ear, Bilateral
Antrum of Highmore (syn)	Maxillary Sinus, Right
Antrum of Highmore (syn)	Maxillary Sinus, Left
Aortic annulus	Aortic Valve
Aortic arch (syn)	Thoracic Aorta
Aortic intercostal artery	Thoracic Aorta
Apical (subclavicular) lymph node	Lymphatic, Left Axillary
Apical (subclavicular) lymph node	Lymphatic, Right Axillary
Apneustic center	Pons
Aqueduct of Sylvius	Cerebral Ventricle
Aqueous humour	Anterior Chamber, Right
Aqueous humour	Anterior Chamber, Left
Arachnoid mater	Cerebral Meninges
Arachnoid mater	Spinal Meninges
Arcuate artery	Foot Artery, Right
Arcuate artery	Foot Artery, Right
Areola	Nipple, Left
Areola	Nipple, Right
Aryepiglottic fold	Larynx
Arytenoid cartilage	Larynx
Arytenoid muscle	Neck Muscle, Right
Arytenoid muscle	Neck Muscle, Left
Arytenoid tendon	Head and Neck Tendon
Ascending aorta (syn)	Thoracic Aorta
Ascending palatine artery	Face Artery
Ascending pharyngeal artery	External Carotid Artery, Right
Ascending pharyngeal artery	External Carotid Artery, Left
Atlantoaxial joint	Cervical Vertebral Joint
Atrioventricular node	Conduction Mechanism
Atrium dextrum cordis (syn)	Atrium, Right
Atrium pulmonale (syn)	Atrium, Left
Auditory tube (syn)	Eustachian Tube, Right
Auditory tube (syn)	Eustachian Tube, Left
Auerbach's (myenteric) plexus	Abdominal Sympathetic Nerve

ICD-10 PROCEDURE CODING SYSTEM
MEDICAL/SURGICAL SECTION
BODY PART KEY BY ANATOMICAL TERM

Anatomical Term	PCS Description
Auricle	External Ear, Right
Auricle	External Ear, Left
Auricle	External Ear, Bilateral
Auricularis tendon	Head and Neck Tendon
Auricularis muscle	Head Muscle
Axillary fascia	Subcutaneous Tissue and Fascia, Right Upper Arm
Axillary fascia	Subcutaneous Tissue and Fascia, Left Upper Arm
Axillary nerve	Brachial Plexus
Bartholin's (greater vestibular) gland	Vestibular Gland
Basal (internal) cerebral vein	Intracranial Vein
Basal nuclei (syn)	Basal Ganglia
Basilar artery	Intracranial Artery
Basis pontis	Pons
Biceps brachii muscle	Upper Arm Muscle, Right
Biceps brachii muscle	Upper Arm Muscle, Left
Biceps brachii tendon	Upper Arm Tendon, Right
Biceps brachii tendon	Upper Arm Tendon, Left
Biceps femoris muscle	Upper Leg Muscle, Right
Biceps femoris muscle	Upper Leg Muscle, Left
Biceps femoris tendon	Upper Leg Tendon, Right
Biceps femoris tendon	Upper Leg Tendon, Left
Bicipital aponeurosis	Subcutaneous Tissue and Fascia, Right Lower Arm
Bicipital aponeurosis	Subcutaneous Tissue and Fascia, Left Lower Arm
Bicuspid valve (syn)	Mitral Valve
Body of femur (syn)	Femoral Shaft, Right
Body of femur (syn)	Femoral Shaft, Left
Body of fibula	Fibula, Left
Body of fibula	Fibula, Right
Bony labyrinth (syn)	Inner Ear, Left
Bony labyrinth (syn)	Inner Ear, Right
Bony orbit (syn)	Orbit, Left
Bony orbit (syn)	Orbit, Right
Bony vestibule	Inner Ear, Left
Bony vestibule	Inner Ear, Right
Brachial (lateral) lymph node	Lymphatic, Left Axillary
Brachial (lateral) lymph node	Lymphatic, Right Axillary
Brachialis muscle	Upper Arm Muscle, Right
Brachialis muscle	Upper Arm Muscle, Left

ICD-10 PROCEDURE CODING SYSTEM
MEDICAL/SURGICAL SECTION
BODY PART KEY BY ANATOMICAL TERM

Anatomical Term	PCS Description
Brachialis tendon	Upper Arm Tendon, Right
Brachialis tendon	Upper Arm Tendon, Left
Brachiocephalic trunk (syn)	Innominate Artery
Brachiocephalic artery (syn)	Innominate Artery
Brachiocephalic vein (syn)	Innominate Vein, Right
Brachiocephalic vein (syn)	Innominate Vein, Left
Brachioradialis tendon	Lower Arm and Wrist Tendon, Right
Brachioradialis tendon	Lower Arm and Wrist Tendon, Left
Brachioradialis muscle	Lower Arm and Wrist Muscle, Right
Brachioradialis muscle	Lower Arm and Wrist Muscle, Left
Broad ligament	Uterine Supporting Structure
Bronchial artery	Thoracic Aorta
Buccal gland	Buccal Mucosa
Buccinator lymph node	Lymphatic, Head
Buccinator muscle	Facial Muscle
Bulbospongiosus muscle	Perineum Muscle
Bulbospongiosus tendon	Perineum Tendon
Bulbourethral (Cowper's) gland	Urethra
Bundle of His	Conduction Mechanism
Bundle of Kent	Conduction Mechanism
Calcaneocuboid ligament	Foot Bursa and Ligament, Right
Calcaneocuboid ligament	Foot Bursa and Ligament, Left
Calcaneocuboid joint	Tarsal Joint, Right
Calcaneocuboid joint	Tarsal Joint, Left
Calcaneofibular ligament	Ankle Bursa and Ligament, Right
Calcaneofibular ligament	Ankle Bursa and Ligament, Left
Calcaneus	Tarsal, Left
Calcaneus	Tarsal, Right
Capitate bone	Carpal, Left
Capitate bone	Carpal, Right
Cardia (syn)	Esophagogastric Junction
Cardiac plexus	Thoracic Sympathetic Nerve
Cardioesophageal junction (syn)	Esophagogastric Junction
Caroticotympanic artery	Internal Carotid Artery, Right
Caroticotympanic artery	Internal Carotid Artery, Left
Carotid glomus (syn)	Carotid Bodies, Bilateral
Carotid glomus (syn)	Carotid Body, Right
Carotid glomus (syn)	Carotid Body, Left
Carotid sinus nerve	Glossopharyngeal Nerve
Carotid sinus (syn)	Internal Carotid Artery, Right
Carotid sinus (syn)	Internal Carotid Artery, Left
Carpometacarpal ligament	Hand Bursa and Ligament, Right

ICD-10 PROCEDURE CODING SYSTEM
MEDICAL/SURGICAL SECTION
BODY PART KEY BY ANATOMICAL TERM

Anatomical Term	PCS Description
Carpometacarpal ligament	Hand Bursa and Ligament, Left
Carpometacarpal (CMC) joint (syn)	Metacarpocarpal Joint, Right
Carpometacarpal (CMC) joint (syn)	Metacarpocarpal Joint, Left
Cauda equina	Lumbar Spinal Cord
Cavernous plexus	Head and Neck Sympathetic Nerve
Celiac (solar) plexus	Abdominal Sympathetic Nerve
Celiac ganglion	Abdominal Sympathetic Nerve
Celiac lymph node	Lymphatic, Aortic
Celiac trunk (syn)	Celiac Artery
Central axillary lymph node	Lymphatic, Left Axillary
Central axillary lymph node	Lymphatic, Right Axillary
Cerebral aqueduct (Sylvius)	Cerebral Ventricle
Cerebrum (syn)	Brain
Cervical esophagus (syn)	Esophagus, Upper
Cervical facet joint	Cervical Vertebral Joints, 2 or more
Cervical facet joint	Cervical Vertebral Joint
Cervical ganglion	Head and Neck Sympathetic Nerve
Cervical intertransverse ligament	Head and Neck Bursa and Ligament
Cervical interspinous ligament	Head and Neck Bursa and Ligament
Cervical ligamentum flavum	Head and Neck Bursa and Ligament
Cervical lymph node	Lymphatic, Left Neck
Cervical lymph node	Lymphatic, Right Neck
Cervicothoracic facet joint	Cervicothoracic Vertebral Joint
Choana	Nasopharynx
Chondroglossus muscle	Tongue, Palate, Pharynx Muscle
Chorda tympani	Facial Nerve
Choroid plexus	Cerebral Ventricle
Ciliary body	Eye, Left
Ciliary body	Eye, Right
Ciliary ganglion	Head and Neck Sympathetic Nerve
Circle of Willis	Intracranial Artery
Circumflex illiac artery	Femoral Artery, Right
Circumflex iliac artery	Femoral Artery, Left
Claustrum	Basal Ganglia
Coccygeal body (syn)	Coccygeal Glomus
Coccygeus muscle	Trunk Muscle, Left
Coccygeus tendon	Trunk Tendon, Left
Cochlea	Inner Ear, Left
Cochlea	Inner Ear, Right
Cochlear nerve	Acoustic Nerve
Columella	Nose
Common digital vein	Foot Vein, Left

ICD-10 PROCEDURE CODING SYSTEM
MEDICAL/SURGICAL SECTION
BODY PART KEY BY ANATOMICAL TERM

Anatomical Term	PCS Description
Common digital vein	Foot Vein, Right
Common facial vein	Face Vein, Left
Common facial vein	Face Vein, Right
Common fibular nerve (syn)	Peroneal Nerve
Common hepatic artery (syn)	Hepatic Artery
Common iliac (subaortic) lymph node	Lymphatic, Pelvis
Common interosseous artery	Ulnar Artery, Right
Common interosseous artery	Ulnar Artery, Left
Common peroneal nerve (syn)	Peroneal Nerve
Condyloid process	Mandible, Left
Condyloid process	Mandible, Right
Conus arteriosus	Ventricle, Right
Conus medullaris	Lumbar Spinal Cord
Coracoacromial ligament	Shoulder Bursa and Ligament, Right
Coracoacromial ligament	Shoulder Bursa and Ligament, Left
Coracobrachialis muscle	Upper Arm Muscle, Right
Coracobrachialis muscle	Upper Arm Muscle, Left
Coracobrachialis tendon	Upper Arm Tendon, Right
Coracobrachialis tendon	Upper Arm Tendon, Left
Coracoclavicular ligament	Shoulder Bursa and Ligament, Right
Coracoclavicular ligament	Shoulder Bursa and Ligament, Left
Coracohumeral ligament	Shoulder Bursa and Ligament, Right
Coracohumeral ligament	Shoulder Bursa and Ligament, Left
Coracoid process	Scapula, Left
Coracoid process	Scapula, Right
Corniculate cartilage	Larynx
Corpus callosum	Brain
Corpus cavernosum	Penis
Corpus spongiosum	Penis
Corpus striatum	Basal Ganglia
Corrugator supercilii muscle	Facial Muscle
Costocervical trunk	Subclavian Artery, Right
Costocervical trunk	Subclavian Artery, Left
Costoclavicular ligament	Shoulder Bursa and Ligament, Right
Costoclavicular ligament	Shoulder Bursa and Ligament, Left
Costotransverse joint	Thoracic Vertebral Joints, 8 or more
Costotransverse joint	Thoracic Vertebral Joints, 2 to 7
Costotransverse joint	Thoracic Vertebral Joint
Costotransverse ligament	Thorax Bursa and Ligament, Right
Costotransverse ligament	Thorax Bursa and Ligament, Left
Costovertebral joint	Thoracic Vertebral Joints, 8 or more
Costovertebral joint	Thoracic Vertebral Joints, 2 to 7

ICD-10 PROCEDURE CODING SYSTEM
MEDICAL/SURGICAL SECTION
BODY PART KEY BY ANATOMICAL TERM

Anatomical Term	PCS Description
Costovertebral joint	Thoracic Vertebral Joint
Costoxiphoid ligament	Thorax Bursa and Ligament, Right
Costoxiphoid ligament	Thorax Bursa and Ligament, Left
Cowper's (bulbourethral) gland	Urethra
Cranial dura mater	Dura Mater
Cranial epidural space	Epidural Space
Cranial subarachnoid space	Subarachnoid Space
Cranial subdural space	Subdural Space
Cremaster muscle	Perineum Muscle
Cremaster tendon	Perineum Tendon
Cribriform plate	Ethmoid Bone, Right
Cribriform plate	Ethmoid Bone, Left
Cricoid cartilage	Larynx
Cricothyroid tendon	Head and Neck Tendon
Cricothyroid muscle	Neck Muscle, Right
Cricothyroid muscle	Neck Muscle, Left
Cricothyroid artery	Thyroid Artery, Right
Cricothyroid artery	Thyroid Artery, Left
Crural fascia	Subcutaneous Tissue and Fascia, Right Upper Leg
Crural fascia	Subcutaneous Tissue and Fascia, Left Upper Leg
Cubital lymph node	Lymphatic, Left Upper Extremity
Cubital lymph node	Lymphatic, Right Upper Extremity
Cubital nerve (syn)	Ulnar Nerve
Cuboid bone	Tarsal, Left
Cuboid bone	Tarsal, Right
Cuboideonavicular joint	Tarsal Joint, Right
Cuboideonavicular joint	Tarsal Joint, Left
Culmen (syn)	Cerebellum
Cuneiform cartilage	Larynx
Cuneonavicular ligament	Foot Bursa and Ligament, Right
Cuneonavicular ligament	Foot Bursa and Ligament, Left
Cuneonavicular joint	Tarsal Joint, Right
Cuneonavicular joint	Tarsal Joint, Left
Cutaneous (transverse) cervical nerve	Cervical Plexus
Deep cervical fascia	Subcutaneous Tissue and Fascia, Anterior Neck
Deep cervical vein	Vertebral Vein, Right
Deep cervical vein	Vertebral Vein, Left
Deep circumflex iliac artery	External Iliac Artery, Right
Deep circumflex Iliac artery	External Iliac Artery, Left

ICD-10 PROCEDURE CODING SYSTEM
MEDICAL/SURGICAL SECTION
BODY PART KEY BY ANATOMICAL TERM

Anatomical Term	PCS Description
Deep facial vein	Face Vein, Left
Deep facial vein	Face Vein, Right
Deep femoral artery	Femoral Artery, Right
Deep femoral artery	Femoral Artery, Left
Deep femoral (profunda femoris) vein	Femoral Vein, Right
Deep femoral (profunda femoris) vein	Femoral Vein, Left
Deep palmar arch	Hand Artery, Right
Deep palmar arch	Hand Artery, Left
Deep transverse perineal muscle	Perineum Muscle
Deep transverse perineal tendon	Perineum Tendon
Deferential artery	Internal Iliac Artery, Right
Deferential artery	Internal Iliac Artery, Left
Deltoid fascia	Subcutaneous Tissue and Fascia, Right Upper Arm
Deltoid fascia	Subcutaneous Tissue and Fascia, Left Upper Arm
Deltoid ligament	Ankle Bursa and Ligament, Right
Deltoid ligament	Ankle Bursa and Ligament, Left
Deltoid muscle	Shoulder Muscle, Right
Deltoid muscle	Shoulder Muscle, Left
Deltoid tendon	Shoulder Tendon, Right
Deltoid tendon	Shoulder Tendon, Left
Deltopectoral (infraclavicular) lymph node	Lymphatic, Left Upper Extremity
Deltopectoral (infraclavicular) lymph node	Lymphatic, Right Upper Extremity
Dentate ligament	Dura Mater
Denticulate ligament	Spinal Cord
Depressor anguli oris muscle	Facial Muscle
Depressor labii inferioris muscle	Facial Muscle
Depressor septi nasi muscle	Facial Muscle
Depressor supercilii muscle	Facial Muscle
Dermis	Skin
Descending genicular artery	Femoral Artery, Right
Descending genicular artery	Femoral Artery, Left
Diaphragma sellae	Dura Mater
Distal radioulnar joint	Wrist Joint, Right
Distal radioulnar joint	Wrist Joint, Left
Dorsal digital nerve	Radial Nerve
Dorsal metacarpal vein	Hand Vein, Left
Dorsal metacarpal vein	Hand Vein, Right
Dorsal metatarsal artery	Foot Artery, Right
Dorsal metatarsal artery	Foot Artery, Left
Dorsal metatarsal vein	Foot Vein, Left

ICD-10 PROCEDURE CODING SYSTEM
MEDICAL/SURGICAL SECTION
BODY PART KEY BY ANATOMICAL TERM

Anatomical Term	PCS Description
Dorsal metatarsal vein	Foot Vein, Right
Dorsal scapular nerve	Brachial Plexus
Dorsal scapular artery	Subclavian Artery, Right
Dorsal scapular artery	Subclavian Artery, Left
Dorsal venous arch	Foot Vein, Left
Dorsal venous arch	Foot Vein, Right
Dorsalis pedis artery	Anterior Tibial Artery, Right
Dorsalis pedis artery	Anterior Tibial Artery, Left
Duct of Santorini (syn)	Pancreatic Duct, Accessory
Duct of Wirsung (syn)	Pancreatic Duct
Ductus deferens (syn)	Vas Deferens, Right
Ductus deferens (syn)	Vas Deferens, Left
Ductus deferens (syn)	Vas Deferens, Bilateral
Ductus deferens (syn)	Vas Deferens
Duodenal ampulla (syn)	Ampulla of Vater
Duodenojejunal flexure	Jejunum
Dural venous sinus	Intracranial Vein
Earlobe	External Ear, Right
Earlobe	External Ear, Left
Earlobe	External Ear, Bilateral
Eighth cranial nerve (syn)	Acoustic Nerve
Ejaculatory duct	Vas Deferens, Right
Ejaculatory duct	Vas Deferens, Left
Ejaculatory duct	Vas Deferens, Bilateral
Ejaculatory duct	Vas Deferens
Eleventh cranial nerve (syn)	Accessory Nerve
Encephalon	Brain
Ependyma (syn)	Cerebral Ventricle
Epidermis	Skin
Epiploic foramen	Peritoneum
Epithalamus	Thalamus
Epitroclear lymph node	Lymphatic, Left Upper Extremity
Epitroclear lymph node	Lymphatic, Right Upper Extremity
Erector spinae muscle	Trunk Muscle, Right
Erector spinae muscle	Trunk Muscle, Left
Erector spinae tendon	Trunk Tendon, Right
Erector spinae tendon	Trunk Tendon, Left
Esophageal artery	Thoracic Aorta
Esophageal plexus	Thoracic Sympathetic Nerve
Ethmoidal air cell (syn)	Ethmoid Sinus, Right
Ethmoidal air cell (syn)	Ethmoid Sinus, Left
Extensor carpi ulnaris tendon	Lower Arm and Wrist Tendon, Right

ICD-10 PROCEDURE CODING SYSTEM
MEDICAL/SURGICAL SECTION
BODY PART KEY BY ANATOMICAL TERM

Anatomical Term	PCS Description
Extensor carpi radialis tendon	Lower Arm and Wrist Tendon, Right
Extensor carpi ulnaris	Lower Arm and Wrist Tendon, Left
Extensor carpi radialis	Lower Arm and Wrist Tendon, Left
Extensor carpi ulnaris muscle	Lower Arm and Wrist Muscle, Right
Extensor carpi radialis muscle	Lower Arm and Wrist Muscle, Right
Extensor carpi ulnaris	Lower Arm and Wrist Muscle, Left
Extensor carpi radialis	Lower Arm and Wrist Muscle, Left
Extensor digitorum brevis muscle	Foot Muscle, Right
Extensor digitorum brevis muscle	Foot Muscle, Left
Extensor digitorum brevis tendon	Foot Tendon, Right
Extensor digitorum brevis tendon	Foot Tendon, Left
Extensor digitorum longus muscle	Lower Leg Muscle, Right
Extensor digitorum longus muscle	Lower Leg Muscle, Left
Extensor digitorum longus tendon	Lower Leg Tendon, Right
Extensor digitorum longus tendon	Lower Leg Tendon, Left
Extensor hallucis brevis muscle	Foot Muscle, Right
Extensor hallucis brevis muscle	Foot Muscle, Left
Extensor hallucis brevis tendon	Foot Tendon, Right
Extensor hallucis brevis tendon	Foot Tendon, Left
Extensor hallucis longus muscle	Lower Leg Muscle, Right
Extensor hallucis longus muscle	Lower Leg Muscle, Left
Extensor hallucis longus tendon	Lower Leg Tendon, Right
Extensor hallucis longus tendon	Lower Leg Tendon, Left
External anal sphincter	Anal Sphincter
External auditory meatus (syn)	External Auditory Canal, Right
External auditory meatus (syn)	External Auditory Canal, Left
External maxillary artery (syn)	Face Artery
External naris	Nose
External oblique muscle	Abdomen Muscle, Right
External oblique muscle	Abdomen Muscle, Left
External oblique tendon	Abdomen Tendon, Right
External oblique tendon	Abdomen Tendon, Left
External oblique aponeurosis	Subcutaneous Tissue and Fascia, Trunk
External popliteal nerve (syn)	Peroneal Nerve
External pudendal artery	Femoral Artery, Right
External pudendal artery	Femoral Artery, Left
External Pudendal vein	Greater Saphenous Vein, Right
External pudendal vein	Greater Saphenous Vein, Left
External urethral sphincter	Urethra
Extradural space	Epidural Space
Facial artery (syn)	Face Artery
False vocal cord	Larynx

ICD-10 PROCEDURE CODING SYSTEM
MEDICAL/SURGICAL SECTION
BODY PART KEY BY ANATOMICAL TERM

Anatomical Term	PCS Description
Falx cerebri	Dura Mater
Fascia lata	Subcutaneous Tissue and Fascia, Right Upper Leg
Fascia lata	Subcutaneous Tissue and Fascia, Left Upper Leg
Femoral head	Upper Femur, Right
Femoral head	Upper Femur, Left
Femoral lymph node	Lymphatic, Left Lower Extremity
Femoral lymph node	Lymphatic, Right Lower Extremity
Femoropatellar joint	Knee Joint, Right
Femoropatellar joint	Knee Joint, Left
Femorotibial joint	Knee Joint, Right
Femorotibial joint	Knee Joint, Left
Fibular artery (syn)	Peroneal Artery, Right
Fibular artery (syn)	Peroneal Artery, Left
Fibularis brevis muscle	Lower Leg Muscle, Right
Fibularis brevis muscle	Lower Leg Muscle, Left
Fibularis brevis tendon	Lower Leg Tendon, Right
Fibularis brevis tendon	Lower Leg Tendon, Left
Fibularis longus muscle	Lower Leg Muscle, Right
Fibularis longus muscle	Lower Leg Muscle, Left
Fibularis longus tendon	Lower Leg Tendon, Right
Fibularis longus tendon	Lower Leg Tendon, Left
Fifth cranial nerve (syn)	Trigeminal Nerve
First cranial nerve (syn)	Olfactory Nerve
First intercostal nerve	Brachial Plexus
Flexor carpi ulnaris tendon	Lower Arm and Wrist Tendon, Right
Flexor carpi radialis tendon	Lower Arm and Wrist Tendon, Right
Flexor carpi ulnaris tendon	Lower Arm and Wrist Tendon, Left
Flexor carpi radialis tendon	Lower Arm and Wrist Tendon, Left
Flexor carpi ulnaris muscle	Lower Arm and Wrist Muscle, Right
Flexor carpi radialis muscle	Lower Arm and Wrist Muscle, Right
Flexor carpi ulnaris muscle	Lower Arm and Wrist Muscle, Left
Flexor carpi radialis muscle	Lower Arm and Wrist Muscle, Left
Flexor digitorum brevis muscle	Foot Muscle, Right
Flexor digitorum brevis muscle	Foot Muscle, Left
Flexor digitorum brevis tendon	Foot Tendon, Right
Flexor digitorum brevis tendon	Foot Tendon, Left
Flexor digitorum longus muscle	Lower Leg Muscle, Right
Flexor digitorum longus muscle	Lower Leg Muscle, Left
Flexor digitorum longus tendon	Lower Leg Tendon, Right
Flexor digitorum longus tendon	Lower Leg Tendon, Left

ICD-10 PROCEDURE CODING SYSTEM
MEDICAL/SURGICAL SECTION
BODY PART KEY BY ANATOMICAL TERM

Anatomical Term	PCS Description
Flexor hallucis brevis muscle	Foot Muscle, Right
Flexor hallucis brevis muscle	Foot Muscle, Left
Flexor hallucis brevis tendon	Foot Tendon, Right
Flexor hallucis brevis tendon	Foot Tendon, Left
Flexor hallucis longus muscle	Lower Leg Muscle, Right
Flexor hallucis longus muscle	Lower Leg Muscle, Left
Flexor hallucis longus tendon	Lower Leg Tendon, Right
Flexor hallucis longus tendon	Lower Leg Tendon, Left
Flexor pollicis longus tendon	Lower Arm and Wrist Tendon, Right
Flexor pollicis longus tendon	Lower Arm and Wrist Tendon, Left
Flexor pollicis longus muscle	Lower Arm and Wrist Muscle, Right
Flexor pollicis longus muscle	Lower Arm and Wrist Muscle, Left
Foramen magnum	Occipital Bone, Right
Foramen magnum	Occipital Bone, Left
Foramen of Monro (intraventricular)	Cerebral Ventricle
Foreskin	Prepuce
Fossa of Rosenmuller	Nasopharynx
Fourth cranial nerve (syn)	Trochlear Nerve
Fourth ventricle	Cerebral Ventricle
Fovea	Retina, Left
Fovea	Retina, Right
Frenulum labii inferioris	Lower Lip
Frenulum labii superioris	Upper Lip
Frenulum linguae	Tongue
Frontal lobe	Cerebral Hemisphere
Frontal vein	Face Vein, Left
Frontal vein	Face Vein, Right
Fundus uteri	Uterus
Galea aponeurotica	Subcutaneous Tissue and Fascia, Scalp
Ganglion impar (ganglion of Walther)	Sacral Sympathetic Nerve
Gasserian ganglion	Trigeminal Nerve
Gastric lymph node	Lymphatic, Aortic
Gastric plexus	Abdominal Sympathetic Nerve
Gastrocnemius muscle	Lower Leg Muscle, Right
Gastrocnemius muscle	Lower Leg Muscle, Left
Gastrocnemius tendon	Lower Leg Tendon, Right
Gastrocnemius tendon	Lower Leg Tendon, Left
Gastrocolic omentum (syn)	Greater Omentum
Gastrocolic ligament	Greater Omentum
Gastroduodenal artery	Hepatic Artery
Gastroesophageal (GE) junction (syn)	Esophagogastric Junction
Gastrohepatic omentum (syn)	Lesser Omentum

ICD-10 PROCEDURE CODING SYSTEM
MEDICAL/SURGICAL SECTION
BODY PART KEY BY ANATOMICAL TERM

Anatomical Term	PCS Description
Gastrophrenic ligament	Greater Omentum
Gastrosplenic ligament	Greater Omentum
Gemellus muscle	Hip Muscle, Right
Gemellus muscle	Hip Muscle, Left
Gemellus tendon	Hip Tendon, Right
Gemellus tendon	Hip Tendon, Left
Geniculate ganglion	Facial Nerve
Geniculate nucleus	Thalamus
Genioglossus muscle	Tongue, Palate, Pharynx Muscle
Genitofemoral nerve	Lumbar Plexus
Glans penis (syn)	Prepuce
Glenohumeral ligament	Shoulder Bursa and Ligament, Right
Glenohumeral ligament	Shoulder Bursa and Ligament, Left
Glenohumeral joint (syn)	Shoulder Joint, Right
Glenohumeral joint (syn)	Shoulder Joint, Left
Glenoid fossa (of scapula) (syn)	Glenoid Cavity, Right
Glenoid fossa (of scapula) (syn)	Glenoid Cavity, Left
Glenoid ligament (labrum)	Shoulder Bursa and Ligament, Right
Glenoid ligament (labrum)	Shoulder Bursa and Ligament, Left
Globus pallidus	Basal Ganglia
Glossoepiglottic fold	Epiglottis
Glottis	Larynx
Gluteal lymph node	Lymphatic, Pelvis
Gluteal vein	Hypogastric Vein, Right
Gluteal vein	Hypogastric Vein, Left
Gluteus maximus muscle	Hip Muscle, Right
Gluteus maximus muscle	Hip Muscle, Left
Gluteus maximus tendon	Hip Tendon, Right
Gluteus maximus tendon	Hip Tendon, Left
Gluteus medius muscle	Hip Muscle, Right
Gluteus medius muscle	Hip Muscle, Left
Gluteus medius tendon	Hip Tendon, Right
Gluteus medius tendon	Hip Tendon, Left
Gluteus minimus muscle	Hip Muscle, Right
Gluteus minimus muscle	Hip Muscle, Left
Gluteus minimus tendon	Hip Tendon, Right
Gluteus minimus tendon	Hip Tendon, Left
Gracilis muscle	Upper Leg Muscle, Right
Gracilis muscle	Upper Leg Muscle, Left
Gracilis tendon	Upper Leg Tendon, Right
Gracilis tendon	Upper Leg Tendon, Left
Great auricular nerve	Cervical Plexus

ICD-10 PROCEDURE CODING SYSTEM
MEDICAL/SURGICAL SECTION
BODY PART KEY BY ANATOMICAL TERM

Anatomical Term	PCS Description
Great cerebral vein	Intracranial Vein
Great saphenous vein (syn)	Greater Saphenous Vein, Right
Great saphenous vein (syn)	Greater Saphenous Vein, Left
Greater alar cartilage	Nose
Greater occipital nerve	Cervical Nerve
Greater splanchnic nerve	Thoracic Sympathetic Nerve
Greater superficial petrosal nerve	Facial Nerve
Greater trochanter	Upper Femur, Right
Greater trochanter	Upper Femur, Left
Greater tuberosity	Humeral Head, Right
Greater tuberosity	Humeral Head, Left
Greater vestibular (Bartholin's) gland	Vestibular Gland
Greater wing	Sphenoid Bone, Right
Greater wing	Sphenoid Bone, Left
Hallux	1st Toe, Left
Hallux	1st Toe, Right
Hamate bone	Carpal, Left
Hamate bone	Carpal, Right
Head of fibula	Fibula, Left
Head of fibula	Fibula, Right
Helix	External Ear, Right
Helix	External Ear, Left
Helix	External Ear, Bilateral
Hepatic artery proper	Hepatic Artery
Hepatic flexure	Ascending Colon
Hepatic lymph node	Lymphatic, Aortic
Hepatic plexus	Abdominal Sympathetic Nerve
Hepatic portal vein (syn)	Portal Vein
Hepatogastric ligament	Lesser Omentum
Hepatopancreatic ampulla (syn)	Ampulla of Vater
Humeroradial joint	Elbow Joint, Right
Humeroradial joint	Elbow Joint, Left
Humeroulnar joint	Elbow Joint, Right
Humeroulnar joint	Elbow Joint, Left
Hyoglossus muscle	Tongue, Palate, Pharynx Muscle
Hyoid artery	Thyroid Artery, Right
Hyoid artery	Thyroid Artery, Left
Hypogastric artery (syn)	Internal Iliac Artery, Right
Hypogastric artery (syn)	Internal Iliac Artery, Left
Hypopharynx	Pharynx
Hypophysis (syn)	Pituitary Gland
Hypothenar muscle	Hand Muscle, Right

ICD-10 PROCEDURE CODING SYSTEM
MEDICAL/SURGICAL SECTION
BODY PART KEY BY ANATOMICAL TERM

Anatomical Term	PCS Description
Hypothenar muscle	Hand Muscle, Left
Hypothenar tendon	Hand Tendon, Right
Hypothenar tendon	Hand Tendon, Left
Ileal artery	Superior Mesenteric Artery
Ileocolic artery	Superior Mesenteric Artery
Ileocolic vein	Colic Vein
Iliac crest	Pelvic Bone, Right
Iliac crest	Pelvic Bone, Left
Iliac fascia	Subcutaneous Tissue and Fascia, Right Upper Leg
Iliac fascia	Subcutaneous Tissue and Fascia, Left Upper Leg
Iliac lymph node	Lymphatic, Pelvis
Iliacus muscle	Hip Muscle, Right
Iliacus muscle	Hip Muscle, Left
Iliacus tendon	Hip Tendon, Right
Iliacus tendon	Hip Tendon, Left
Iliofemoral ligament	Hip Bursa and Ligament, Right
Iliofemoral ligament	Hip Bursa and Ligament, Left
Iliohypogastric nerve	Lumbar Plexus
Ilioinguinal nerve	Lumbar Plexus
Iliolumbar artery	Internal Iliac Artery, Right
Iliolumbar artery	Internal Iliac Artery, Left
Iliolumbar ligament	Trunk Bursa and Ligament, Right
Iliolumbar ligament	Trunk Bursa and Ligament, Left
Iliotibial tract (band)	Subcutaneous Tissue and Fascia, Right Upper Leg
Iliotibial tract (band)	Subcutaneous Tissue and Fascia, Left Upper Leg
Ilium	Pelvic Bone, Right
Ilium	Pelvic Bone, Left
Incus	Auditory Ossicle, Right
Incus	Auditory Ossicle, Left
Inferior cardiac nerve	Thoracic Sympathetic Nerve
Inferior cerebral vein	Intracranial Vein
Inferior cerebellar vein	Intracranial Vein
Inferior epigastric artery	External Iliac Artery, Right
Inferior epigastric artery	External Iliac Artery, Left
Inferior epigastric lymph node	Lymphatic, Pelvis
Inferior genicular artery	Popliteal Artery, Right
Inferior genicular artery	Popliteal Artery, Left
Inferior gluteal artery	Internal Iliac Artery, Right

ICD-10 PROCEDURE CODING SYSTEM
MEDICAL/SURGICAL SECTION
BODY PART KEY BY ANATOMICAL TERM

Anatomical Term	PCS Description
Inferior gluteal artery	Internal Iliac Artery, Left
Inferior gluteal nerve	Sacral Plexus
Inferior hypogastric plexus	Abdominal Sympathetic Nerve
Inferior labial artery	Face Artery
Inferior longitudinal muscle	Tongue, Palate, Pharynx Muscle
Inferior mesenteric plexus	Abdominal Sympathetic Nerve
Inferior mesenteric ganglion	Abdominal Sympathetic Nerve
Inferior mesenteric lymph node	Lymphatic, Mesenteric
Inferior oblique muscle	Extraocular Muscle, Right
Inferior oblique muscle	Extraocular Muscle, Left
Inferior pancreaticoduodenal artery	Superior Mesenteric Artery
Inferior phrenic artery	Abdominal Aorta
Inferior rectus muscle	Extraocular Muscle, Right
Inferior rectus muscle	Extraocular Muscle, Left
Inferior suprarenal artery	Renal Artery, Right
Inferior suprarenal artery	Renal Artery, Left
Inferior tarsal plate	Lower Eyelid, Right
Inferior tarsal plate	Lower Eyelid, Left
Inferior thyroid vein	Innominate Vein, Right
Inferior thyroid vein	Innominate Vein, Left
Inferior tibiofibular joint	Ankle Joint, Right
Inferior tibiofibular joint	Ankle Joint, Left
Inferior turbinate	Nasal Turbinate
Inferior ulnar collateral artery	Brachial Artery, Right
Inferior ulnar collateral artery	Brachial Artery, Left
Inferior vesical artery	Internal Iliac Artery, Right
Inferior vesical artery	Internal Iliac Artery, Left
Infraauricular lymph node	Lymphatic, Head
Infraclavicular (deltopectoral) lymph node	Lymphatic, Left Upper Extremity
Infraclavicular (deltopectoral) lymph node	Lymphatic, Right Upper Extremity
Infrahyoid muscle	Neck Muscle, Right
Infrahyoid muscle	Neck Muscle, Left
Infrahyoid tendon	Head and Neck Tendon
Infraparotid lymph node	Lymphatic, Head
Infraspinatus muscle	Shoulder Muscle, Right
Infraspinatus muscle	Shoulder Muscle, Left
Infraspinatus tendon	Shoulder Tendon, Right
Infraspinatus tendon	Shoulder Tendon, Left
Infraspinatus fascia	Subcutaneous Tissue and Fascia, Right Upper Arm
Infraspinatus fascia	Subcutaneous Tissue and Fascia, Left Upper Arm

ICD-10 PROCEDURE CODING SYSTEM
MEDICAL/SURGICAL SECTION
BODY PART KEY BY ANATOMICAL TERM

Anatomical Term	PCS Description
Infundibulopelvic ligament	Uterine Supporting Structure
Inguinal canal	Inguinal Region, Right
Inguinal canal	Inguinal Region, Left
Inguinal canal	Inguinal Region, Bilateral
Inguinal triangle (syn)	Inguinal Region, Right
Inguinal triangle (syn)	Inguinal Region, Left
Inguinal triangle (syn)	Inguinal Region, Bilateral
Interatrial septum (syn)	Atrial Septum
Interatrial septum	Heart
Intercarpal joint	Carpal Joint, Right
Intercarpal joint	Carpal Joint, Left
Intercarpal ligament	Hand Bursa and Ligament, Right
Intercarpal ligament	Hand Bursa and Ligament, Left
Interclavicular ligament	Shoulder Bursa and Ligament, Right
Interclavicular ligament	Shoulder Bursa and Ligament, Left
Intercostal lymph node	Lymphatic, Thorax
Intercostal nerve	Thoracic Nerve
Intercostal muscle	Thorax Muscle, Right
Intercostal muscle	Thorax Muscle, Left
Intercostal tendon	Thorax Tendon, Right
Intercostal tendon	Thorax Tendon, Left
Intercostobrachial nerve	Thoracic Nerve
Intercuneiform ligament	Foot Bursa and Ligament, Right
Intercuneiform ligament	Foot Bursa and Ligament, Left
Intercuneiform joint	Tarsal Joint, Right
Intercuneiform joint	Tarsal Joint, Left
Intermediate cuneiform bone	Tarsal, Left
Intermediate cuneiform bone	Tarsal, Right
Internal (basal) cerebral vein	Intracranial Vein
Internal anal sphincter	Anal Sphincter
Internal carotid plexus	Head and Neck Sympathetic Nerve
Internal iliac vein (syn)	Hypogastric Vein, Right
Internal iliac vein (syn)	Hypogastric Vein, Left
Internal maxillary artery	External Carotid Artery, Right
Internal maxillary artery	External Carotid Artery, Left
Internal naris	Nose
Internal oblique muscle	Abdomen Muscle, Right
Internal oblique muscle	Abdomen Muscle, Left
Internal oblique tendon	Abdomen Tendon, Right
Internal oblique tendon	Abdomen Tendon, Left
Internal pudendal vein	Hypogastric Vein, Right
Internal pudendal vein	Hypogastric Vein, Left

ICD-10 PROCEDURE CODING SYSTEM
MEDICAL/SURGICAL SECTION
BODY PART KEY BY ANATOMICAL TERM

Anatomical Term	PCS Description
Internal pudendal artery	Internal Iliac Artery, Right
Internal pudendal artery	Internal Iliac Artery, Left
Internal thoracic artery (syn)	Internal Mammary Artery, Right
Internal thoracic artery (syn)	Internal Mammary Artery, Left
Internal thoracic artery	Subclavian Artery, Right
Internal thoracic artery	Subclavian Artery, Left
Internal urethral sphincter	Urethra
Interphalangeal (IP) joint (syn)	Finger Phalangeal Joint, Right
Interphalangeal (IP) joint (syn)	Finger Phalangeal Joint, Left
Interphalangeal ligament	Foot Bursa and Ligament, Right
Interphalangeal ligament	Foot Bursa and Ligament, Left
Interphalangeal ligament	Hand Bursa and Ligament, Right
Interphalangeal ligament	Hand Bursa and Ligament, Left
Interphalangeal (IP) joint (syn)	Toe Phalangeal Joint, Right
Interphalangeal (IP) joint (syn)	Toe Phalangeal Joint, Left
Interspinalis muscle	Trunk Muscle, Right
Interspinalis muscle	Trunk Muscle, Left
Interspinalis tendon	Trunk Tendon, Right
Interspinalis tendon	Trunk Tendon, Left
Interspinous ligament	Trunk Bursa and Ligament, Right
Interspinous ligament	Trunk Bursa and Ligament, Left
Intertransverse ligament	Trunk Bursa and Ligament, Right
Intertransverse ligament	Trunk Bursa and Ligament, Left
Intertransversarius muscle	Trunk Muscle, Right
Intertransversarius muscle	Trunk Muscle, Left
Intertransversarius tendon	Trunk Tendon, Right
Intertransversarius tendon	Trunk Tendon, Left
Interventricular foramen (Monro)	Cerebral Ventricle
Interventricular septum (syn)	Ventricular Septum
Intestinal lymphatic trunk	Cisterna Chyli
Ischiatic nerve (syn)	Sciatic Nerve
Ischiocavernosus muscle	Perineum Muscle
Ischiocavernosus tendon	Perineum Tendon
Ischiofemoral ligament	Hip Bursa and Ligament, Right
Ischiofemoral ligament	Hip Bursa and Ligament, Left
Ischium	Pelvic Bone, Right
Ischium	Pelvic Bone, Left
Jejunal artery	Superior Mesenteric Artery
Jugular body (syn)	Glomus Jugulare
Jugular lymph node	Lymphatic, Left Neck
Jugular lymph node	Lymphatic, Right Neck
Labia majora	Vulva

ICD-10 PROCEDURE CODING SYSTEM
MEDICAL/SURGICAL SECTION
BODY PART KEY BY ANATOMICAL TERM

Anatomical Term	PCS Description
Labia minora	Vulva
Labial gland	Buccal Mucosa
Lacrimal canaliculus	Lacrimal Duct, Right
Lacrimal canaliculus	Lacrimal Duct, Left
Lacrimal punctum	Lacrimal Duct, Right
Lacrimal punctum	Lacrimal Duct, Left
Lacrimal sac	Lacrimal Duct, Right
Lacrimal sac	Lacrimal Duct, Left
Laryngopharynx	Pharynx
Lateral (brachial) lymph node	Lymphatic, Left Axillary
Lateral (brachial) lymph node	Lymphatic, Right Axillary
Lateral canthus	Upper Eyelid, Right
Lateral canthus	Upper Eyelid, Left
Lateral collateral ligament (LCL)	Knee Bursa and Ligament, Right
Lateral collateral ligament (LCL)	Knee Bursa and Ligament, Left
Lateral condyle of femur	Lower Femur, Right
Lateral condyle of femur	Lower Femur, Left
Lateral condyle of tibia	Tibia, Left
Lateral condyle of tibia	Tibia, Right
Lateral cuneiform bone	Tarsal, Left
Lateral cuneiform bone	Tarsal, Right
Lateral epicondyle of humerus	Humeral Shaft, Right
Lateral epicondyle of humerus	Humeral Shaft, Left
Lateral epicondyle of femur	Lower Femur, Right
Lateral epicondyle of femur	Lower Femur, Left
Lateral femoral cutaneous nerve	Lumbar Plexus
Lateral malleolus	Fibula, Left
Lateral malleolus	Fibula, Right
Lateral meniscus	Knee Joint, Right
Lateral meniscus	Knee Joint, Left
Lateral nasal cartilage	Nose
Lateral plantar artery	Foot Artery, Right
Lateral plantar artery	Foot Artery, Left
Lateral plantar nerve	Tibial Nerve
Lateral rectus muscle	Extraocular Muscle, Right
Lateral rectus muscle	Extraocular Muscle, Left
Lateral sacral vein	Hypogastric Vein, Right
Lateral sacral vein	Hypogastric Vein, Left
Lateral sacral artery	Internal Iliac Artery, Right
Lateral sacral artery	Internal Iliac Artery, Left
Lateral sural cutaneous nerve	Peroneal Nerve
Lateral tarsal artery	Foot Artery, Right

ICD-10 PROCEDURE CODING SYSTEM
MEDICAL/SURGICAL SECTION
BODY PART KEY BY ANATOMICAL TERM

Anatomical Term	PCS Description
Lateral tarsal artery	Foot Artery, Right
Lateral temporomandibular ligament	Head and Neck Bursa and Ligament
Lateral thoracic artery	Axillary Artery, Right
Lateral thoracic artery	Axillary Artery, Left
Latissimus dorsi muscle	Trunk Muscle, Right
Latissimus dorsi muscle	Trunk Muscle, Left
Latissimus dorsi tendon	Trunk Tendon, Right
Latissimus dorsi tendon	Trunk Tendon, Left
Least splanchnic nerve	Thoracic Sympathetic Nerve
Left ascending lumbar vein	Hemiazygos Vein
Left atrioventricular valve (syn)	Mitral Valve
Left auricular appendix	Atrium, Left
Left colic vein	Colic Vein
Left coronary sulcus	Heart, Left
Left gastric artery	Gastric Artery
Left gastroepiploic artery	Splenic Artery
Left gastroepiploic vein	Splenic Vein
Left Inferior pulmonary vein	Pulmonary Vein, Left
Left inferior phrenic vein	Renal Vein, Left
Left jugular trunk	Thoracic Duct
Left lateral ventricle	Cerebral Ventricle
Left ovarian vein	Renal Vein, Left
Left second lumbar vein	Renal Vein, Left
Left subclavian trunk	Thoracic Duct
Left subcostal vein	Hemiazygos Vein
Left superior pulmonary vein	Pulmonary Vein, Left
Left suprarenal vein	Renal Vein, Left
Left testicular vein	Renal Vein, Left
Leptomeninges	Cerebral Meninges
Leptomeninges	Spinal Meninges
Lesser alar cartilage	Nose
Lesser occipital nerve	Cervical Plexus
Lesser splanchnic nerve	Thoracic Sympathetic Nerve
Lesser trochanter	Upper Femur, Right
Lesser trochanter	Upper Femur, Left
Lesser tuberosity	Humeral Head, Right
Lesser tuberosity	Humeral Head, Left
Lesser wing	Sphenoid Bone, Right
Lesser wing	Sphenoid Bone, Left
Levator anguli oris muscle	Facial Muscle
Levator ani muscle	Trunk Muscle, Left
Levator ani tendon	Trunk Tendon, Left

ICD-10 PROCEDURE CODING SYSTEM
MEDICAL/SURGICAL SECTION
BODY PART KEY BY ANATOMICAL TERM

Anatomical Term	PCS Description
Levator labii superioris muscle	Facial Muscle
Levator labii superioris alaeque nasi muscle	Facial Muscle
Levator palpebrae superioris muscle	Upper Eyelid, Right
Levator palpebrae superioris muscle	Upper Eyelid, Left
Levator scapulae tendon	Head and Neck Tendon
Levator scapulae muscle	Neck Muscle, Right
Levator scapulae muscle	Neck Muscle, Left
Levator veli palatini muscle	Tongue, Palate, Pharynx Muscle
Levatores costarum muscle	Thorax Muscle, Right
Levatores costarum muscle	Thorax Muscle, Left
Levatores costarum tendon	Thorax Tendon, Right
Levatores costarum tendon	Thorax Tendon, Left
Ligament of the lateral malleolus	Ankle Bursa and Ligament, Right
Ligament of the lateral malleolus	Ankle Bursa and Ligament, Left
Ligament of head of fibula	Knee Bursa and Ligament, Right
Ligament of head of fibula	Knee Bursa and Ligament, Left
Ligamentum flavum	Trunk Bursa and Ligament, Right
Ligamentum flavum	Trunk Bursa and Ligament, Left
Lingual artery	External Carotid Artery, Right
Lingual artery	External Carotid Artery, Left
Lingual tonsil	Tongue
Locus ceruleus	Pons
Long thoracic nerve	Brachial Plexus
Lumbar artery	Abdominal Aorta
Lumbar facet joint	Lumbar Vertebral Joints, 2 or more
Lumbar facet joint	Lumbar Vertebral Joint
Lumbar ganglion	Lumbar Sympathetic Nerve
Lumbar lymphatic trunk	Cisterna Chyli
Lumbar lymph node	Lymphatic, Aortic
Lumbar splanchnic nerve	Lumbar Sympathetic Nerve
Lumbosacral trunk	Lumbar Nerve
Lumbosacral facet joint	Lumbosacral Joint
Lunate bone	Carpal, Left
Lunate bone	Carpal, Right
Lunotriquetral ligament	Hand Bursa and Ligament, Right
Lunotriquetral ligament	Hand Bursa and Ligament, Left
Macula	Retina, Left
Macula	Retina, Right
Malleus	Auditory Ossicle, Right
Malleus	Auditory Ossicle, Left
Mammary duct	Breast, Bilateral
Mammary duct	Breast, Left

ICD-10 PROCEDURE CODING SYSTEM
MEDICAL/SURGICAL SECTION
BODY PART KEY BY ANATOMICAL TERM

Anatomical Term	PCS Description
Mammary duct	Breast, Right
Mammary gland	Breast, Bilateral
Mammary gland	Breast, Left
Mammary gland	Breast, Right
Mammillary body	Hypothalamus
Mandibular notch	Mandible, Left
Mandibular notch	Mandible, Right
Mandibular nerve	Trigeminal Nerve
Manubrium	Sternum
Masseter muscle	Head Muscle
Masseter tendon	Head and Neck Tendon
Masseteric fascia	Subcutaneous Tissue and Fascia, Face
Mastoid (postauricular) lymph node	Lymphatic, Left Neck
Mastoid (postauricular) lymph node	Lymphatic, Right Neck
Mastoid air cells	Mastoid Sinus, Right
Mastoid air cells	Mastoid Sinus, Left
Mastoid process	Temporal Bone, Right
Mastoid process	Temporal Bone, Left
Maxillary artery	External Carotid Artery, Right
Maxillary artery	External Carotid Artery, Left
Maxillary nerve	Trigeminal Nerve
Medial canthus	Lower Eyelid, Right
Medial canthus	Lower Eyelid, Left
Medial collateral ligament (MCL)	Knee Bursa and Ligament, Right
Medial collateral ligament (MCL)	Knee Bursa and Ligament, Left
Medial condyle of femur	Lower Femur, Right
Medial condyle of femur	Lower Femur, Left
Medial condyle of tibia	Tibia, Left
Medial condyle of tibia	Tibia, Right
Medial cuneiform bone	Tarsal, Left
Medial cuneiform bone	Tarsal, Right
Medial epicondyle of humerus	Humeral Shaft, Right
Medial epicondyle of humerus	Humeral Shaft, Left
Medial epicondyle of femur	Lower Femur, Right
Medial epicondyle of femur	Lower Femur, Left
Medial malleolus	Tibia, Left
Medial malleolus	Tibia, Right
Medial meniscus	Knee Joint, Right
Medial meniscus	Knee Joint, Left
Medial plantar artery	Foot Artery, Right
Medial plantar artery	Foot Artery, Left
Medial plantar nerve	Tibial Nerve

ICD-10 PROCEDURE CODING SYSTEM
MEDICAL/SURGICAL SECTION
BODY PART KEY BY ANATOMICAL TERM

Anatomical Term	PCS Description
Medial popliteal nerve	Tibial Nerve
Medial rectus muscle	Extraocular Muscle, Right
Medial rectus muscle	Extraocular Muscle, Left
Medial sural cutaneous nerve	Tibial Nerve
Median antebrachial vein	Basilic Vein, Right
Median antebrachial vein	Basilic Vein, Left
Median cubital vein	Basilic Vein, Right
Median cubital vein	Basilic Vein, Left
Median sacral artery	Abdominal Aorta
Mediastinal lymph node	Lymphatic, Thorax
Meissner's (submucous) plexus	Abdominal Sympathetic Nerve
Membranous urethra	Urethra
Mental foramen	Mandible, Left
Mental foramen	Mandible, Right
Mentalis muscle	Facial Muscle
Mesoappendix	Mesentery
Mesocolon	Mesentery
Metacarpal ligament	Hand Bursa and Ligament, Right
Metacarpal ligament	Hand Bursa and Ligament, Left
Metacarpophalangeal ligament	Hand Bursa and Ligament, Right
Metacarpophalangeal ligament	Hand Bursa and Ligament, Left
Metatarsal ligament	Foot Bursa and Ligament, Right
Metatarsal ligament	Foot Bursa and Ligament, Left
Metatarsophalangeal ligament	Foot Bursa and Ligament, Right
Metatarsophalangeal ligament	Foot Bursa and Ligament, Left
Metatarsophalangeal (MTP) joint (syn)	Metatarsal-Phalangeal Joint, Right
Metatarsophalangeal (MTP) joint (syn)	Metatarsal-Phalangeal Joint, Left
Metathalamus	Thalamus
Midcarpal joint	Carpal Joint, Right
Midcarpal joint	Carpal Joint, Left
Middle cardiac nerve	Thoracic Sympathetic Nerve
Middle cerebral artery	Intracranial Artery
Middle cerebral vein	Intracranial Vein
Middle colic vein	Colic Vein
Middle genicular artery	Popliteal Artery, Right
Middle genicular artery	Popliteal Artery, Left
Middle hemorrhoidal vein	Hypogastric Vein, Right
Middle hemorrhoidal vein	Hypogastric Vein, Left
Middle rectal artery	Internal Iliac Artery, Right
Middle rectal artery	Internal Iliac Artery, Left
Middle suprarenal artery	Abdominal Aorta
Middle temporal artery	Temporal Artery, Right

ICD-10 PROCEDURE CODING SYSTEM
MEDICAL/SURGICAL SECTION
BODY PART KEY BY ANATOMICAL TERM

Anatomical Term	PCS Description
Middle temporal artery	Temporal Artery, Left
Middle turbinate	Nasal Turbinate
Mitral annulus	Mitral Valve
Molar gland	Buccal Mucosa
Musculocutaneous nerve	Brachial Plexus
Musculophrenic artery	Internal Mammary Artery, Right
Musculophrenic artery	Internal Mammary Artery, Left
Musculospiral nerve	Radial Nerve
Myelencephalon (syn)	Medulla Oblongata
Myenteric (Auerbach's) plexus	Abdominal Sympathetic Nerve
Myometrium	Uterus
Nail bed	Finger Nail
Nail bed	Toe Nail
Nail plate	Finger Nail
Nail plate	Toe Nail
Nasal cavity	Nose
Nasal concha (syn)	Nasal Turbinate
Nasalis muscle	Facial Muscle
Nasolacrimal duct	Lacrimal Duct, Right
Nasolacrimal duct	Lacrimal Duct, Left
Navicular bone	Tarsal, Left
Navicular bone	Tarsal, Right
Neck of femur	Upper Femur, Right
Neck of femur	Upper Femur, Left
Neck of humerus (anatomical)(surgical)	Humeral Head, Right
Neck of humerus (anatomical)(surgical)	Humeral Head, Left
Nerve to the stapedius	Facial Nerve
Neurohypophysis	Pituitary Gland
Ninth cranial nerve (syn)	Glossopharyngeal Nerve
Nostril	Nose
Obturator artery	Internal Iliac Artery, Right
Obturator artery	Internal Iliac Artery, Left
Obturator lymph node	Lymphatic, Pelvis
Obturator muscle	Hip Muscle, Right
Obturator muscle	Hip Muscle, Left
Obturator nerve	Lumbar Plexus
Obturator tendon	Hip Tendon, Right
Obturator tendon	Hip Tendon, Left
Obturator vein	Hypogastric Vein, Right
Obturator vein	Hypogastric Vein, Left
Obtuse margin	Heart, Left
Occipital artery	External Carotid Artery, Right

ICD-10 PROCEDURE CODING SYSTEM
MEDICAL/SURGICAL SECTION
BODY PART KEY BY ANATOMICAL TERM

Anatomical Term	PCS Description
Occipital artery	External Carotid Artery, Left
Occipital lobe	Cerebral Hemisphere
Occipital lymph node	Lymphatic, Left Neck
Occipital lymph node	Lymphatic, Right Neck
Occipitofrontalis muscle	Facial Muscle
Olecranon bursa	Elbow Bursa and Ligament, Right
Olecranon bursa	Elbow Bursa and Ligament, Left
Olecranon process	Ulna, Left
Olecranon process	Ulna, Right
Olfactory bulb	Olfactory Nerve
Ophthalmic artery	Internal Carotid Artery, Right
Ophthalmic artery	Internal Carotid Artery, Left
Ophthalmic nerve	Trigeminal Nerve
Ophthalmic vein	Intracranial Vein
Optic chiasma	Optic Nerve
Optic disc	Retina, Left
Optic disc	Retina, Right
Optic foramen	Sphenoid Bone, Right
Optic foramen	Sphenoid Bone, Left
Orbicularis oris muscle	Facial Muscle
Orbicularis oculi muscle	Upper Eyelid, Right
Orbicularis oculi muscle	Upper Eyelid, Left
Orbital fascia	Subcutaneous Tissue and Fascia, Face
Orbital portion of zygomatic bone	Orbit, Left
Orbital portion of sphenoid bone	Orbit, Left
Orbital portion of palatine bone	Orbit, Left
Orbital portion of maxilla	Orbit, Left
Orbital portion of lacrimal bone	Orbit, Left
Orbital portion of frontal bone	Orbit, Left
Orbital portion of ethmoid bone	Orbit, Left
Orbital portion of zygomatic bone	Orbit, Right
Orbital portion of sphenoid bone	Orbit, Right
Orbital portion of palatine bone	Orbit, Right
Orbital portion of maxilla	Orbit, Right
Orbital portion of lacrimal bone	Orbit, Right
Orbital portion of frontal bone	Orbit, Right
Orbital portion of ethmoid bone	Orbit, Right
Oropharynx	Pharynx
Ossicular chain	Auditory Ossicle, Right
Ossicular chain	Auditory Ossicle, Left
Otic ganglion	Head and Neck Sympathetic Nerve
Oval window	Inner Ear, Left

ICD-10 PROCEDURE CODING SYSTEM
MEDICAL/SURGICAL SECTION
BODY PART KEY BY ANATOMICAL TERM

Anatomical Term	PCS Description
Oval window	Inner Ear, Right
Ovarian artery	Abdominal Aorta
Ovarian ligament	Uterine Supporting Structure
Oviduct (syn)	Fallopian Tube, Right
Oviduct (syn)	Fallopian Tube, Left
Palatine gland	Buccal Mucosa
Palatine tonsil	Tonsils
Palatine uvula (syn)	Uvula
Palatoglossal muscle	Tongue, Palate, Pharynx Muscle
Palatopharyngeal muscle	Tongue, Palate, Pharynx Muscle
Palmar (volar) metacarpal vein	Hand Vein, Left
Palmar (volar) digital vein	Hand Vein, Left
Palmar (volar) metacarpal vein	Hand Vein, Right
Palmar (volar) digital vein	Hand Vein, Right
Palmar cutaneous nerve	Median Nerve
Palmar cutaneous nerve	Radial Nerve
Palmar fascia (aponeurosis)	Subcutaneous Tissue and Fascia, Right Hand
Palmar fascia (aponeurosis)	Subcutaneous Tissue and Fascia, Left Hand
Palmar interosseous muscle	Hand Muscle, Right
Palmar interosseous muscle	Hand Muscle, Left
Palmar interosseous tendon	Hand Tendon, Right
Palmar interosseous tendon	Hand Tendon, Left
Palmar ulnocarpal ligament	Wrist Bursa and Ligament, Right
Palmar ulnocarpal ligament	Wrist Bursa and Ligament, Left
Palmaris longus tendon	Lower Arm and Wrist Tendon, Right
Palmaris longus tendon	Lower Arm and Wrist Tendon, Left
Palmaris longus muscle	Lower Arm and Wrist Muscle, Right
Palmaris longus muscle	Lower Arm and Wrist Muscle, Left
Pancreatic artery	Splenic Artery
Pancreatic plexus	Abdominal Sympathetic Nerve
Pancreatic vein	Splenic Vein
Pancreaticosplenic lymph node	Lymphatic, Aortic
Paraaortic lymph node (syn)	Lymphatic, Aortic
Pararectal lymph node	Lymphatic, Mesenteric
Parasternal lymph node	Lymphatic, Thorax
Paratracheal lymph node	Lymphatic, Thorax
Paraurethral (Skene's) gland	Vestibular Gland
Parietal lobe	Cerebral Hemisphere
Parotid lymph node	Lymphatic, Head
Parotid plexus	Facial Nerve

ICD-10 PROCEDURE CODING SYSTEM
MEDICAL/SURGICAL SECTION
BODY PART KEY BY ANATOMICAL TERM

Anatomical Term	PCS Description
Pars flaccida	Tympanic Membrane, Right
Pars flaccida	Tympanic Membrane, Left
Patellar ligament	Knee Bursa and Ligament, Right
Patellar ligament	Knee Bursa and Ligament, Left
Patellar tendon	Knee Tendon, Right
Patellar tendon	Knee Tendon, Left
Pectineus muscle	Upper Leg Muscle, Right
Pectineus muscle	Upper Leg Muscle, Left
Pectineus tendon	Upper Leg Tendon, Right
Pectineus tendon	Upper Leg Tendon, Left
Pectoral (anterior) lymph node	Lymphatic, Left Axillary
Pectoral (anterior) lymph node	Lymphatic, Right Axillary
Pectoral fascia	Subcutaneous Tissue and Fascia, Chest
Pectoralis minor muscle	Thorax Muscle, Right
Pectoralis major muscle	Thorax Muscle, Right
Pectoralis minor muscle	Thorax Muscle, Left
Pectoralis major muscle	Thorax Muscle, Left
Pectoralis minor tendon	Thorax Tendon, Right
Pectoralis major tendon	Thorax Tendon, Right
Pectoralis minor tendon	Thorax Tendon, Left
Pectoralis major tendon	Thorax Tendon, Left
Pelvic fascia	Subcutaneous Tissue and Fascia, Trunk
Pelvic splanchnic nerve	Abdominal Sympathetic Nerve
Pelvic splanchnic nerve	Sacral Sympathetic Nerve
Penile urethra	Urethra
Pericardiophrenic artery	Internal Mammary Artery, Right
Pericardiophrenic artery	Internal Mammary Artery, Left
Perimetrium	Uterus
Peroneus brevis muscle	Lower Leg Muscle, Right
Peroneus brevis muscle	Lower Leg Muscle, Left
Peroneus brevis tendon	Lower Leg Tendon, Right
Peroneus brevis tendon	Lower Leg Tendon, Left
Peroneus longus muscle	Lower Leg Muscle, Right
Peroneus longus muscle	Lower Leg Muscle, Left
Peroneus longus tendon	Lower Leg Tendon, Right
Peroneus longus tendon	Lower Leg Tendon, Left
Petrous part of temoporal bone	Temporal Bone, Right
Petrous part of temoporal bone	Temporal Bone, Left
Pharyngeal constrictor muscle	Tongue, Palate, Pharynx Muscle
Pharyngeal plexus	Vagus Nerve
Pharyngeal recess	Nasopharynx
Pharyngeal tonsil	Adenoids

ICD-10 PROCEDURE CODING SYSTEM
MEDICAL/SURGICAL SECTION
BODY PART KEY BY ANATOMICAL TERM

Anatomical Term	PCS Description
Pharyngotympanic tube (syn)	Eustachian Tube, Right
Pharyngotympanic tube (syn)	Eustachian Tube, Left
Pia mater	Cerebral Meninges
Pia mater	Spinal Meninges
Pinna (syn)	External Ear, Right
Pinna (syn)	External Ear, Left
Pinna (syn)	External Ear, Bilateral
Piriform recess (sinus)	Pharynx
Piriformis muscle	Hip Muscle, Right
Piriformis muscle	Hip Muscle, Left
Piriformis tendon	Hip Tendon, Right
Piriformis tendon	Hip Tendon, Left
Pisiform bone	Carpal, Left
Pisiform bone	Carpal, Right
Pisohamate ligament	Hand Bursa and Ligament, Right
Pisohamate ligament	Hand Bursa and Ligament, Left
Pisometacarpal ligament	Hand Bursa and Ligament, Right
Pisometacarpal ligament	Hand Bursa and Ligament, Left
Plantar digital vein	Foot Vein, Left
Plantar digital vein	Foot Vein, Right
Plantar fascia (aponeurosis)	Subcutaneous Tissue and Fascia, Right Foot
Plantar fascia (aponeurosis)	Subcutaneous Tissue and Fascia, Left Foot
Plantar metatarsal vein	Foot Vein, Left
Plantar metatarsal vein	Foot Vein, Right
Plantar venous arch	Foot Vein, Left
Plantar venous arch	Foot Vein, Right
Platysma muscle	Neck Muscle, Right
Platysma muscle	Neck Muscle, Left
Platysma tendon	Head and Neck Tendon
Plica semilunaris	Conjunctiva, Right
Plica semilunaris	Conjunctiva, Left
Pneumogastric nerve (syn)	Vagus Nerve
Pneumotaxic center	Pons
Pontine tegmentum	Pons
Popliteal lymph node	Lymphatic, Left Lower Extremity
Popliteal lymph node	Lymphatic, Right Lower Extremity
Popliteal ligament	Knee Bursa and Ligament, Right
Popliteal ligament	Knee Bursa and Ligament, Left
Popliteal vein	Femoral Vein, Right
Popliteal vein	Femoral Vein, Left

ICD-10 PROCEDURE CODING SYSTEM
MEDICAL/SURGICAL SECTION
BODY PART KEY BY ANATOMICAL TERM

Anatomical Term	PCS Description
Popliteus muscle	Lower Leg Muscle, Right
Popliteus muscle	Lower Leg Muscle, Left
Popliteus tendon	Lower Leg Tendon, Right
Popliteus tendon	Lower Leg Tendon, Left
Postauricular (mastoid) lymph node	Lymphatic, Left Neck
Postauricular (mastoid) lymph node	Lymphatic, Right Neck
Postcava (syn)	Inferior Vena Cava
Posterior (subscapular) lymph node	Lymphatic, Left Axillary
Posterior (subscapular) lymph node	Lymphatic, Right Axillary
Posterior auricular artery	External Carotid Artery, Right
Posterior auricular artery	External Carotid Artery, Left
Posterior auricular vein	External Jugular Vein, Right
Posterior auricular vein	External Jugular Vein, Left
Posterior auricular nerve	Facial Nerve
Posterior cerebral artery	Intracranial Artery
Posterior chamber	Eye, Left
Posterior chamber	Eye, Right
Posterior circumflex humeral artery	Axillary Artery, Right
Posterior circumflex humeral artery	Axillary Artery, Left
Posterior communicating artery	Intracranial Artery
Posterior cruciate ligament (PCL)	Knee Bursa and Ligament, Right
Posterior cruciate ligament (PCL)	Knee Bursa and Ligament, Left
Posterior facial (retromandibular) vein	Face Vein, Left
Posterior facial (retromandibular) vein	Face Vein, Right
Posterior femoral cutaneous nerve	Sacral Plexus
Posterior inferior cerebellar artery (PICA)	Intracranial Artery
Posterior interosseous nerve	Radial Nerve
Posterior labial nerve	Pudendal Nerve
Posterior scrotal nerve	Pudendal Nerve
Posterior spinal artery	Vertebral Artery, Right
Posterior spinal artery	Vertebral Artery, Left
Posterior tibial recurrent artery	Anterior Tibial Artery, Right
Posterior tibial recurrent artery	Anterior Tibial Artery, Left
Posterior ulnar recurrent artery	Ulnar Artery, Right
Posterior ulnar recurrent artery	Ulnar Artery, Left
Posterior vagal trunk	Vagus Nerve
Preauricular lymph node	Lymphatic, Head
Precava (syn)	Superior Vena Cava
Prepatellar bursa	Knee Bursa and Ligament, Right
Prepatellar bursa	Knee Bursa and Ligament, Left
Pretracheal fascia	Subcutaneous Tissue and Fascia, Anterior Neck

ICD-10 PROCEDURE CODING SYSTEM
MEDICAL/SURGICAL SECTION
BODY PART KEY BY ANATOMICAL TERM

Anatomical Term	PCS Description
Prevertebral fascia	Subcutaneous Tissue and Fascia, Posterior Neck
Princeps pollicis artery	Hand Artery, Right
Princeps pollicis artery	Hand Artery, Left
Procerus muscle	Facial Muscle
Profunda brachii	Brachial Artery, Right
Profunda brachii	Brachial Artery, Left
Profunda femoris (deep femoral) vein	Femoral Vein, Right
Profunda femoris (deep femoral) vein	Femoral Vein, Left
Pronator quadratus tendon	Lower Arm and Wrist Tendon, Right
Pronator quadratus tendon	Lower Arm and Wrist Tendon, Left
Pronator quadratus muscle	Lower Arm and Wrist Muscle, Right
Pronator quadratus muscle	Lower Arm and Wrist Muscle, Left
Pronator teres tendon	Lower Arm and Wrist Tendon, Right
Pronator teres tendon	Lower Arm and Wrist Tendon, Left
Pronator teres muscle	Lower Arm and Wrist Muscle, Right
Pronator teres muscle	Lower Arm and Wrist Muscle, Left
Prostatic urethra	Urethra
Proximal radioulnar joint	Elbow Joint, Right
Proximal radioulnar joint	Elbow Joint, Left
Psoas muscle	Hip Muscle, Right
Psoas muscle	Hip Muscle, Left
Psoas tendon	Hip Tendon, Right
Psoas tendon	Hip Tendon, Left
Pterygoid muscle	Head Muscle
Pterygoid process	Sphenoid Bone, Right
Pterygoid process	Sphenoid Bone, Left
Pterygoid tendon	Head and Neck Tendon
Pterygopalatine (sphenopalatine) ganglion	Head and Neck Sympathetic Nerve
Pubic ligament	Trunk Bursa and Ligament, Right
Pubic ligament	Trunk Bursa and Ligament, Left
Pubis	Pelvic Bone, Right
Pubis	Pelvic Bone, Left
Pubofemoral ligament	Hip Bursa and Ligament, Right
Pubofemoral ligament	Hip Bursa and Ligament, Left
Pudendal nerve	Sacral Plexus
Pulmonary annulus	Pulmonary Valve
Pulmonary plexus	Thoracic Sympathetic Nerve
Pulmonary plexus	Vagus Nerve
Pulmonic valve (syn)	Pulmonary Valve
Pulvinar	Thalamus
Pyloric antrum	Stomach, Pylorus

ICD-10 PROCEDURE CODING SYSTEM
MEDICAL/SURGICAL SECTION
BODY PART KEY BY ANATOMICAL TERM

Anatomical Term	PCS Description
Pyloric canal	Stomach, Pylorus
Pyloric sphincter	Stomach, Pylorus
Pyramidalis muscle	Abdomen Muscle, Right
Pyramidalis muscle	Abdomen Muscle, Left
Pyramidalis tendon	Abdomen Tendon, Right
Pyramidalis tendon	Abdomen Tendon, Left
Quadrangular cartilage	Nasal Septum
Quadrate lobe	Liver
Quadratus femoris muscle	Hip Muscle, Right
Quadratus femoris muscle	Hip Muscle, Left
Quadratus femoris tendon	Hip Tendon, Right
Quadratus femoris tendon	Hip Tendon, Left
Quadratus lumborum muscle	Trunk Muscle, Right
Quadratus lumborum muscle	Trunk Muscle, Left
Quadratus lumborum tendon	Trunk Tendon, Right
Quadratus lumborum tendon	Trunk Tendon, Left
Quadratus plantae muscle	Foot Muscle, Right
Quadratus plantae muscle	Foot Muscle, Left
Quadratus plantae tendon	Foot Tendon, Right
Quadratus plantae tendon	Foot Tendon, Left
Quadriceps (femoris)	Upper Leg Muscle, Right
Quadriceps (femoris)	Upper Leg Muscle, Left
Quadriceps (femoris)	Upper Leg Tendon, Right
Quadriceps (femoris)	Upper Leg Tendon, Left
Radial collateral ligament	Elbow Bursa and Ligament, Right
Radial collateral ligament	Elbow Bursa and Ligament, Left
Radial collateral carpal ligament	Wrist Bursa and Ligament, Right
Radial collateral carpal ligament	Wrist Bursa and Ligament, Left
Radial notch	Ulna, Left
Radial notch	Ulna, Right
Radial recurrent artery	Radial Artery, Right
Radial recurrent artery	Radial Artery, Left
Radial vein	Brachial Vein, Right
Radial vein	Brachial Vein, Left
Radialis indicis	Hand Artery, Right
Radialis indicis	Hand Artery, Left
Radiocarpal ligament	Wrist Bursa and Ligament, Right
Radiocarpal ligament	Wrist Bursa and Ligament, Left
Radiocarpal joint	Wrist Joint, Right
Radiocarpal joint	Wrist Joint, Left
Radioulnar ligament	Wrist Bursa and Ligament, Right
Radioulnar ligament	Wrist Bursa and Ligament, Left

ICD-10 PROCEDURE CODING SYSTEM
MEDICAL/SURGICAL SECTION
BODY PART KEY BY ANATOMICAL TERM

Anatomical Term	PCS Description
Rectosigmoid junction	Sigmoid Colon
Rectus abdominis muscle	Abdomen Muscle, Right
Rectus abdominis muscle	Abdomen Muscle, Left
Rectus abdominis tendon	Abdomen Tendon, Right
Rectus abdominis tendon	Abdomen Tendon, Left
Rectus femoris muscle	Upper Leg Muscle, Right
Rectus femoris muscle	Upper Leg Muscle, Left
Rectus femoris tendon	Upper Leg Tendon, Right
Rectus femoris tendon	Upper Leg Tendon, Left
Recurrent laryngeal nerve	Vagus Nerve
Renal calyx	Kidney
Renal calyx	Kidney, Left
Renal calyx	Kidney, Right
Renal calyx	Kidneys, Bilateral
Renal capsule	Kidney
Renal capsule	Kidney, Left
Renal capsule	Kidney, Right
Renal capsule	Kidneys, Bilateral
Renal cortex	Kidney
Renal cortex	Kidney, Left
Renal cortex	Kidney, Right
Renal cortex	Kidneys, Bilateral
Renal plexus	Abdominal Sympathetic Nerve
Renal segment	Kidney
Renal segment	Kidney, Left
Renal segment	Kidney, Right
Renal segment	Kidneys, Bilateral
Renal segmental artery	Renal Artery, Right
Renal segmental artery	Renal Artery, Left
Retroperitoneal lymph node	Lymphatic, Aortic
Retroperitoneal space (syn)	Retroperitoneum
Retropharyngeal lymph node	Lymphatic, Left Neck
Retropharyngeal lymph node	Lymphatic, Right Neck
Retropubic space	Pelvic Cavity
Rhinopharynx (syn)	Nasopharynx
Rhomboid major muscle	Trunk Muscle, Right
Rhomboid major muscle	Trunk Muscle, Left
Rhomboid major tendon	Trunk Tendon, Right
Rhomboid major tendon	Trunk Tendon, Left
Rhomboid minor muscle	Trunk Muscle, Right
Rhomboid minor muscle	Trunk Muscle, Left
Rhomboid minor tendon	Trunk Tendon, Right

ICD-10 PROCEDURE CODING SYSTEM
MEDICAL/SURGICAL SECTION
BODY PART KEY BY ANATOMICAL TERM

Anatomical Term	PCS Description
Rhomboid minor tendon	Trunk Tendon, Left
Right ascending lumbar vein	Azygos Vein
Right atrioventricular valve (syn)	Tricuspid Valve
Right auricular appendix	Atrium, Right
Right colic vein	Colic Vein
Right coronary sulcus	Heart, Right
Right gastric artery	Gastric Artery
Right gastroepiploic vein	Superior Mesenteric Vein
Right inferior phrenic vein	Inferior Vena Cava
Right inferior pulmonary vein	Pulmonary Vein, Right
Right jugular trunk	Lymphatic, Right Neck
Right lateral ventricle	Cerebral Ventricle
Right lymphatic duct	Lymphatic, Right Neck
Right ovarian vein	Inferior Vena Cava
Right second lumbar vein	Inferior Vena Cava
Right subclavian trunk	Lymphatic, Right Neck
Right subcostal vein	Azygos Vein
Right superior pulmonary vein	Pulmonary Vein, Right
Right suprarenal vein	Inferior Vena Cava
Right testicular vein	Inferior Vena Cava
Rima glottidis	Larynx
Risorius muscle	Facial Muscle
Round ligament of uterus	Uterine Supporting Structure
Round window	Inner Ear, Left
Round window	Inner Ear, Right
Sacral ganglion	Sacral Sympathetic Nerve
Sacral lymph node	Lymphatic, Pelvis
Sacral splanchnic nerve	Sacral Sympathetic Nerve
Sacrococcygeal symphysis (syn)	Sacrococcygeal Joint
Sacrococcygeal ligament	Trunk Bursa and Ligament, Right
Sacrococcygeal ligament	Trunk Bursa and Ligament, Left
Sacroiliac ligament	Trunk Bursa and Ligament, Right
Sacroiliac ligament	Trunk Bursa and Ligament, Left
Sacrospinous ligament	Trunk Bursa and Ligament, Right
Sacrospinous ligament	Trunk Bursa and Ligament, Left
Sacrotuberous ligament	Trunk Bursa and Ligament, Right
Sacrotuberous ligament	Trunk Bursa and Ligament, Left
Salpingopharyngeus muscle	Tongue, Palate, Pharynx Muscle
Salpinx (syn)	Fallopian Tube, Right
Salpinx (syn)	Fallopian Tube, Left
Saphenous nerve	Femoral Nerve
Sartorius muscle	Upper Leg Muscle, Right

ICD-10 PROCEDURE CODING SYSTEM
MEDICAL/SURGICAL SECTION
BODY PART KEY BY ANATOMICAL TERM

Anatomical Term	PCS Description
Sartorius muscle	Upper Leg Muscle, Left
Sartorius tendon	Upper Leg Tendon, Right
Sartorius tendon	Upper Leg Tendon, Left
Scalene muscle	Neck Muscle, Right
Scalene muscle	Neck Muscle, Left
Scalene tendon	Head and Neck Tendon
Scaphoid bone	Carpal, Left
Scaphoid bone	Carpal, Right
Scapholunate ligament	Hand Bursa and Ligament, Right
Scapholunate ligament	Hand Bursa and Ligament, Left
Scaphotrapezium ligament	Hand Bursa and Ligament, Right
Scaphotrapezium ligament	Hand Bursa and Ligament, Left
Scarpa's (vestibular) ganglion	Acoustic Nerve
Sebaceous gland	Skin
Second cranial nerve (syn)	Optic Nerve
Sella turcica	Sphenoid Bone, Right
Sella turcica	Sphenoid Bone, Left
Semicircular canal	Inner Ear, Left
Semicircular canal	Inner Ear, Right
Semimembranosus muscle	Upper Leg Muscle, Right
Semimembranosus muscle	Upper Leg Muscle, Left
Semimembranosus tendon	Upper Leg Tendon, Right
Semimembranosus tendon	Upper Leg Tendon, Left
Semitendinosus muscle	Upper Leg Muscle, Right
Semitendinosus muscle	Upper Leg Muscle, Left
Semitendinosus tendon	Upper Leg Tendon, Right
Semitendinosus tendon	Upper Leg Tendon, Left
Septal cartilage	Nasal Septum
Serratus anterior muscle	Thorax Muscle, Right
Serratus anterior muscle	Thorax Muscle, Left
Serratus anterior tendon	Thorax Tendon, Right
Serratus anterior tendon	Thorax Tendon, Left
Serratus posterior muscle	Trunk Muscle, Right
Serratus posterior muscle	Trunk Muscle, Left
Serratus posterior tendon	Trunk Tendon, Right
Serratus posterior tendon	Trunk Tendon, Left
Seventh cranial nerve (syn)	Facial Nerve
Short gastric artery	Splenic Artery
Sigmoid artery	Inferior Mesenteric Artery
Sigmoid flexure (syn)	Sigmoid Colon
Sigmoid vein	Inferior Mesenteric Vein
Sinoatrial node	Conduction Mechanism

ICD-10 PROCEDURE CODING SYSTEM
MEDICAL/SURGICAL SECTION
BODY PART KEY BY ANATOMICAL TERM

Anatomical Term	PCS Description
Sinus venosus	Atrium, Right
Sixth cranial nerve (syn)	Abducens Nerve
Skene's (paraurethral) gland	Vestibular Gland
Small saphenous vein (syn)	Lesser Saphenous Vein, Right
Small saphenous vein (syn)	Lesser Saphenous Vein, Left
Solar (celiac) plexus	Abdominal Sympathetic Nerve
Soleus muscle	Lower Leg Muscle, Right
Soleus muscle	Lower Leg Muscle, Left
Soleus tendon	Lower Leg Tendon, Right
Soleus tendon	Lower Leg Tendon, Left
Sphenomandibular ligament	Head and Neck Bursa and Ligament
Sphenopalatine (pterygopalatine) ganglion	Head and Neck Sympathetic Nerve
Spinal dura mater	Dura Mater
Spinal epidural space	Epidural Space
Spinal subarachnoid space	Subarachnoid Space
Spinal subdural space	Subdural Space
Spinous process	Cervical Vertebra
Spinous process	Lumbar Vertebra
Spinous process	Thoracic Vertebra
Spiral ganglion	Acoustic Nerve
Splenic flexure	Transverse Colon
Splenic plexus	Abdominal Sympathetic Nerve
Splenius capitis tendon	Head and Neck Tendon
Splenius capitis muscle	Head Muscle
Splenius cervicis tendon	Head and Neck Tendon
Splenius cervicis muscle	Neck Muscle, Right
Splenius cervicis muscle	Neck Muscle, Left
Stapes	Auditory Ossicle, Right
Stapes	Auditory Ossicle, Left
Stellate ganglion	Head and Neck Sympathetic Nerve
Stensen's duct (syn)	Parotid Duct, Right
Stensen's duct (syn)	Parotid Duct, Left
Sternoclavicular ligament	Shoulder Bursa and Ligament, Right
Sternoclavicular ligament	Shoulder Bursa and Ligament, Left
Sternocleidomastoid tendon	Head and Neck Tendon
Sternocleidomastoid muscle	Neck Muscle, Right
Sternocleidomastoid muscle	Neck Muscle, Left
Sternocleidomastoid artery	Thyroid Artery, Right
Sternocleidomastoid artery	Thyroid Artery, Left
Sternocostal ligament	Thorax Bursa and Ligament, Right
Sternocostal ligament	Thorax Bursa and Ligament, Left
Styloglossus muscle	Tongue, Palate, Pharynx Muscle

ICD-10 PROCEDURE CODING SYSTEM
MEDICAL/SURGICAL SECTION
BODY PART KEY BY ANATOMICAL TERM

Anatomical Term	PCS Description
Stylomandibular ligament	Head and Neck Bursa and Ligament
Stylopharyngeus muscle	Tongue, Palate, Pharynx Muscle
Subacromial bursa	Shoulder Bursa and Ligament, Right
Subacromial bursa	Shoulder Bursa and Ligament, Left
Subaortic (common iliac) lymph node	Lymphatic, Pelvis
Subclavicular (apical) lymph node	Lymphatic, Left Axillary
Subclavicular (apical) lymph node	Lymphatic, Right Axillary
Subclavius muscle	Thorax Muscle, Right
Subclavius muscle	Thorax Muscle, Left
Subclavius nerve	Brachial Plexus
Subclavius tendon	Thorax Tendon, Right
Subclavius tendon	Thorax Tendon, Left
Subcostal artery	Thoracic Aorta
Subcostal muscle	Thorax Muscle, Right
Subcostal muscle	Thorax Muscle, Left
Subcostal nerve	Thoracic Nerve
Subcostal tendon	Thorax Tendon, Right
Subcostal tendon	Thorax Tendon, Left
Submandibular ganglion	Facial Nerve
Submandibular ganglion	Head and Neck Sympathetic Nerve
Submandibular lymph node	Lymphatic, Head
Submandibular gland (syn)	Submaxillary Gland, Right
Submandibular gland (syn)	Submaxillary Gland, Left
Submaxillary ganglion	Head and Neck Sympathetic Nerve
Submaxillary lymph node	Lymphatic, Head
Submental artery	Face Artery
Submental lymph node	Lymphatic, Head
Submucous (Meissner's) plexus	Abdominal Sympathetic Nerve
Suboccipital nerve	Cervical Nerve
Suboccipital venous plexus	Vertebral Vein, Right
Suboccipital venous plexus	Vertebral Vein, Left
Subparotid lymph node	Lymphatic, Head
Subscapular artery	Axillary Artery, Right
Subscapular artery	Axillary Artery, Left
Subscapular (posterior) lymph node	Lymphatic, Left Axillary
Subscapular (posterior) lymph node	Lymphatic, Right Axillary
Subscapular aponeurosis	Subcutaneous Tissue and Fascia, Right Upper Arm
Subscapular aponeurosis	Subcutaneous Tissue and Fascia, Left Upper Arm
Subscapularis muscle	Shoulder Muscle, Right
Subscapularis muscle	Shoulder Muscle, Left

ICD-10 PROCEDURE CODING SYSTEM
MEDICAL/SURGICAL SECTION
BODY PART KEY BY ANATOMICAL TERM

Anatomical Term	PCS Description
Subscapularis tendon	Shoulder Tendon, Right
Subscapularis tendon	Shoulder Tendon, Left
Substantia nigra	Basal Ganglia
Subtalar (talocalcaneal) joint	Tarsal Joint, Right
Subtalar (talocalcaneal) joint	Tarsal Joint, Left
Subtalar ligament	Foot Bursa and Ligament, Right
Subtalar ligament	Foot Bursa and Ligament, Left
Subthalamic nucleus	Basal Ganglia
Superficial epigastric artery	Femoral Artery, Right
Superficial epigastric artery	Femoral Artery, Left
Superficial epigastric vein	Greater Saphenous Vein, Right
Superficial circumflex iliac vein	Greater Saphenous Vein, Right
Superficial epigastric vein	Greater Saphenous Vein, Left
Superficial circumflex iliac vein	Greater Saphenous Vein, Left
Superficial palmar arch	Hand Artery, Right
Superficial palmar arch	Hand Artery, Left
Superficial palmar venous arch	Hand Vein, Left
Superficial palmar venous arch	Hand Vein, Right
Superficial transverse perineal muscle	Perineum Muscle
Superficial transverse perineal tendon	Perineum Tendon
Superficial temporal artery (syn)	Temporal Artery, Right
Superficial temporal artery (syn)	Temporal Artery, Left
Superior cardiac nerve	Thoracic Sympathetic Nerve
Superior cerebral vein	Intracranial Vein
Superior cerebellar vein	Intracranial Vein
Superior clunic (cluneal) nerve	Lumbar Nerve
Superior epigastric artery	Internal Mammary Artery, Right
Superior epigastric artery	Internal Mammary Artery, Left
Superior genicular artery	Popliteal Artery, Right
Superior genicular artery	Popliteal Artery, Left
Superior gluteal artery	Internal Iliac Artery, Right
Superior gluteal artery	Internal Iliac Artery, Left
Superior gluteal nerve	Lumbar Plexus
Superior hypogastric plexus	Abdominal Sympathetic Nerve
Superior labial artery	Face Artery
Superior laryngeal artery	Thyroid Artery, Right
Superior laryngeal artery	Thyroid Artery, Left
Superior laryngeal nerve	Vagus Nerve
Superior longitudinal muscle	Tongue, Palate, Pharynx Muscle
Superior mesenteric plexus	Abdominal Sympathetic Nerve
Superior mesenteric ganglion	Abdominal Sympathetic Nerve
Superior mesenteric lymph node	Lymphatic, Mesenteric

ICD-10 PROCEDURE CODING SYSTEM
MEDICAL/SURGICAL SECTION
BODY PART KEY BY ANATOMICAL TERM

Anatomical Term	PCS Description
Superior oblique muscle	Extraocular Muscle, Right
Superior oblique muscle	Extraocular Muscle, Left
Superior olivary nucleus	Pons
Superior rectus muscle	Extraocular Muscle, Right
Superior rectus muscle	Extraocular Muscle, Left
Superior rectal vein	Inferior Mesenteric Vein
Superior rectal artery	Inferior Mesenteric Artery
Superior tarsal plate	Upper Eyelid, Right
Superior tarsal plate	Upper Eyelid, Left
Superior thoracic artery	Axillary Artery, Right
Superior thoracic artery	Axillary Artery, Left
Superior thyroid artery (syn)	External Carotid Artery, Right
Superior thyroid artery (syn)	External Carotid Artery, Left
Superior thyroid artery (syn)	Thyroid Artery, Right
Superior thyroid artery (syn)	Thyroid Artery, Left
Superior turbinate	Nasal Turbinate
Superior ulnar collateral artery	Brachial Artery, Right
Superior ulnar collateral artery	Brachial Artery, Left
Supraclavicular nerve	Cervical Plexus
Supraclavicular (Virchow's) lymph node	Lymphatic, Left Neck
Supraclavicular (Virchow's) lymph node	Lymphatic, Right Neck
Suprahyoid lymph node	Lymphatic, Head
Suprahyoid muscle	Neck Muscle, Right
Suprahyoid muscle	Neck Muscle, Left
Suprahyoid tendon	Head and Neck Tendon
Suprainguinal lymph node	Lymphatic, Pelvis
Supraorbital vein	Face Vein, Left
Supraorbital vein	Face Vein, Right
Suprarenal gland (syn)	Adrenal Glands, Bilateral
Suprarenal gland (syn)	Adrenal Gland, Right
Suprarenal gland (syn)	Adrenal Gland, Left
Suprarenal gland (syn)	Adrenal Gland
Suprarenal plexus	Abdominal Sympathetic Nerve
Suprascapular nerve	Brachial Plexus
Supraspinatus muscle	Shoulder Muscle, Right
Supraspinatus muscle	Shoulder Muscle, Left
Supraspinatus tendon	Shoulder Tendon, Right
Supraspinatus tendon	Shoulder Tendon, Left
Supraspinatus fascia	Subcutaneous Tissue and Fascia, Right Upper Arm
Supraspinatus fascia	Subcutaneous Tissue and Fascia, Left Upper Arm

ICD-10 PROCEDURE CODING SYSTEM
MEDICAL/SURGICAL SECTION
BODY PART KEY BY ANATOMICAL TERM

Anatomical Term	PCS Description
Supraspinous ligament	Trunk Bursa and Ligament, Right
Supraspinous ligament	Trunk Bursa and Ligament, Left
Suprasternal notch	Sternum
Supratrochlear lymph node	Lymphatic, Left Upper Extremity
Supratrochlear lymph node	Lymphatic, Right Upper Extremity
Sural artery	Popliteal Artery, Right
Sural artery	Popliteal Artery, Left
Sweat gland	Skin
Talocalcaneal ligament	Foot Bursa and Ligament, Right
Talocalcaneal ligament	Foot Bursa and Ligament, Left
Talocalcaneal (subtalar) joint	Tarsal Joint, Right
Talocalcaneal (subtalar) joint	Tarsal Joint, Left
Talocalcaneonavicular ligament	Foot Bursa and Ligament, Right
Talocalcaneonavicular ligament	Foot Bursa and Ligament, Left
Talocalcaneonavicular joint	Tarsal Joint, Right
Talocalcaneonavicular joint	Tarsal Joint, Left
Talocrural joint (syn)	Ankle Joint, Right
Talocrural joint (syn)	Ankle Joint, Left
Talofibular ligament	Ankle Bursa and Ligament, Right
Talofibular ligament	Ankle Bursa and Ligament, Left
Talus bone	Tarsal, Left
Talus bone	Tarsal, Right
Tarsometatarsal ligament	Foot Bursa and Ligament, Right
Tarsometatarsal ligament	Foot Bursa and Ligament, Left
Tarsometatarsal joint (syn)	Metatarsal-Tarsal Joint, Right
Tarsometatarsal joint (syn)	Metatarsal-Tarsal Joint, Left
Temporal lobe	Cerebral Hemisphere
Temporalis muscle	Head Muscle
Temporalis tendon	Head and Neck Tendon
Temporoparietalis tendon	Head and Neck Tendon
Temporoparietalis muscle	Head Muscle
Tensor fasciae latae muscle	Hip Muscle, Right
Tensor fasciae latae	Hip Muscle, Left
Tensor fasciae latae tendon	Hip Tendon, Right
Tensor fasciae latae	Hip Tendon, Left
Tensor veli palatini muscle	Tongue, Palate, Pharynx Muscle
Tenth cranial nerve (syn)	Vagus Nerve
Tentorium cerebelli	Dura Mater
Teres major muscle	Shoulder Muscle, Right
Teres major muscle	Shoulder Muscle, Left
Teres major tendon	Shoulder Tendon, Right
Teres major tendon	Shoulder Tendon, Left

ICD-10 PROCEDURE CODING SYSTEM
MEDICAL/SURGICAL SECTION
BODY PART KEY BY ANATOMICAL TERM

Anatomical Term	PCS Description
Teres minor muscle	Shoulder Muscle, Right
Teres minor muscle	Shoulder Muscle, Left
Teres minor tendon	Shoulder Tendon, Right
Teres minor tendon	Shoulder Tendon, Left
Testicular artery	Abdominal Aorta
Thenar muscle	Hand Muscle, Right
Thenar muscle	Hand Muscle, Left
Thenar tendon	Hand Tendon, Right
Thenar tendon	Hand Tendon, Left
Third cranial nerve (syn)	Oculomotor Nerve
Third occipital nerve	Cervical Nerve
Third ventricle	Cerebral Ventricle
Thoracic aortic plexus	Thoracic Sympathetic Nerve
Thoracic esophagus (syn)	Esophagus, Middle
Thoracic facet joint	Thoracic Vertebral Joints, 8 or more
Thoracic facet joint	Thoracic Vertebral Joints, 2 to 7
Thoracic facet joint	Thoracic Vertebral Joint
Thoracic ganglion	Thoracic Sympathetic Nerve
Thoracoacromial artery	Axillary Artery, Right
Thoracoacromial artery	Axillary Artery, Left
Thoracolumbar facet joint	Thoracolumbar Vertebral Joint
Thymus gland (syn)	Thymus
Thyroarytenoid tendon	Head and Neck Tendon
Thyroarytenoid muscle	Neck Muscle, Right
Thyroarytenoid muscle	Neck Muscle, Left
Thyrocervical trunk (syn)	Thyroid Artery, Right
Thyrocervical trunk (syn)	Thyroid Artery, Left
Thyroid cartilage	Larynx
Tibialis anterior muscle	Lower Leg Muscle, Right
Tibialis anterior muscle	Lower Leg Muscle, Left
Tibialis anterior tendon	Lower Leg Tendon, Right
Tibialis anterior tendon	Lower Leg Tendon, Left
Tibialis posterior muscle	Lower Leg Muscle, Right
Tibialis posterior muscle	Lower Leg Muscle, Left
Tibialis posterior tendon	Lower Leg Tendon, Right
Tibialis posterior tendon	Lower Leg Tendon, Left
Tracheobronchial lymph node	Lymphatic, Thorax
Tragus	External Ear, Right
Tragus	External Ear, Left
Tragus	External Ear, Bilateral
Transversalis fascia	Subcutaneous Tissue and Fascia, Trunk
Transverse (cutaneous) cervical nerve	Cervical Plexus

ICD-10 PROCEDURE CODING SYSTEM
MEDICAL/SURGICAL SECTION
BODY PART KEY BY ANATOMICAL TERM

Anatomical Term	PCS Description
Transverse acetabular ligament	Hip Bursa and Ligament, Right
Transverse acetabular ligament	Hip Bursa and Ligament, Left
Transverse facial artery	Temporal Artery, Right
Transverse facial artery	Temporal Artery, Left
Transverse humeral ligament	Shoulder Bursa and Ligament, Right
Transverse humeral ligament	Shoulder Bursa and Ligament, Left
Transverse ligament of atlas	Head and Neck Bursa and Ligament
Transverse scapular ligament	Shoulder Bursa and Ligament, Right
Transverse scapular ligament	Shoulder Bursa and Ligament, Left
Transverse thoracis muscle	Thorax Muscle, Right
Transverse thoracis muscle	Thorax Muscle, Left
Transverse thoracis tendon	Thorax Tendon, Right
Transverse thoracis tendon	Thorax Tendon, Left
Transversospinalis muscle	Trunk Muscle, Right
Transversospinalis muscle	Trunk Muscle, Left
Transversospinalis tendon	Trunk Tendon, Right
Transversospinalis tendon	Trunk Tendon, Left
Transversus abdominis muscle	Abdomen Muscle, Right
Transversus abdominis muscle	Abdomen Muscle, Left
Transversus abdominis tendon	Abdomen Tendon, Right
Transversus abdominis tendon	Abdomen Tendon, Left
Trapezium bone	Carpal, Left
Trapezium bone	Carpal, Right
Trapezius muscle	Trunk Muscle, Right
Trapezius muscle	Trunk Muscle, Left
Trapezius tendon	Trunk Tendon, Right
Trapezius tendon	Trunk Tendon, Left
Trapezoid bone	Carpal, Left
Trapezoid bone	Carpal, Right
Triceps brachii muscle	Upper Arm Muscle, Right
Triceps brachii muscle	Upper Arm Muscle, Left
Triceps brachii tendon	Upper Arm Tendon, Right
Triceps brachii tendon	Upper Arm Tendon, Left
Tricuspid annulus	Tricuspid Valve
Trifacial nerve (syn)	Trigeminal Nerve
Trigone of bladder	Bladder
Triquetral bone	Carpal, Left
Triquetral bone	Carpal, Right
Trochanteric bursa	Hip Bursa and Ligament, Right
Trochanteric bursa	Hip Bursa and Ligament, Left
Twelfth cranial nerve (syn)	Hypoglossal Nerve
Tympanic cavity (syn)	Middle Ear, Right

ICD-10 PROCEDURE CODING SYSTEM
MEDICAL/SURGICAL SECTION
BODY PART KEY BY ANATOMICAL TERM

Anatomical Term	PCS Description
Tympanic cavity (syn)	Middle Ear, Left
Tympanic nerve	Glossopharyngeal Nerve
Tympanic part of temoporal bone	Temporal Bone, Right
Tympanic part of temoporal bone	Temporal Bone, Left
Ulnar collateral ligament	Elbow Bursa and Ligament, Right
Ulnar collateral ligament	Elbow Bursa and Ligament, Left
Ulnar collateral carpal ligament	Wrist Bursa and Ligament, Right
Ulnar collateral carpal ligament	Wrist Bursa and Ligament, Left
Ulnar notch	Radius, Left
Ulnar notch	Radius, Right
Ulnar vein	Brachial Vein, Right
Ulnar vein	Brachial Vein, Left
Umbilical artery	Internal Iliac Artery, Right
Umbilical artery	Internal Iliac Artery, Left
Ureteral orifice	Ureter
Ureteral orifice	Ureter, Left
Ureteral orifice	Ureter, Right
Ureteral orifice	Ureters, Bilateral
Ureteropelvic junction (UPJ)	Kidney Pelvis, Right
Ureteropelvic junction (UPJ)	Kidney Pelvis, Left
Ureterovesical orifice	Ureter, Left
Ureterovesical orifice	Ureter, Right
Uterine artery	Internal Iliac Artery, Right
Uterine artery	Internal Iliac Artery, Left
Uterine cornu	Uterus
Uterine tube (syn)	Fallopian Tube, Right
Uterine tube (syn)	Fallopian Tube, Left
Uterine vein	Hypogastric Vein, Right
Uterine vein	Hypogastric Vein, Left
Vaginal artery	Internal Iliac Artery, Right
Vaginal artery	Internal Iliac Artery, Left
Vaginal vein	Hypogastric Vein, Right
Vaginal vein	Hypogastric Vein, Left
Vastus intermedius muscle	Upper Leg Muscle, Right
Vastus intermedius muscle	Upper Leg Muscle, Left
Vastus intermedius tendon	Upper Leg Tendon, Right
Vastus intermedius tendon	Upper Leg Tendon, Left
Vastus lateralis muscle	Upper Leg Muscle, Right
Vastus lateralis muscle	Upper Leg Muscle, Left
Vastus lateralis tendon	Upper Leg Tendon, Right
Vastus lateralis tendon	Upper Leg Tendon, Left
Vastus medialis muscle	Upper Leg Muscle, Right

ICD-10 PROCEDURE CODING SYSTEM
MEDICAL/SURGICAL SECTION
BODY PART KEY BY ANATOMICAL TERM

Anatomical Term	PCS Description
Vastus medialis muscle	Upper Leg Muscle, Left
Vastus medialis tendon	Upper Leg Tendon, Right
Vastus medialis tendon	Upper Leg Tendon, Left
Ventricular fold	Larynx
Vermiform appendix (syn)	Appendix
Vermilion border	Lower Lip
Vermilion border	Upper Lip
Vertebral arch	Cervical Vertebra
Vertebral arch	Lumbar Vertebra
Vertebral arch	Thoracic Vertebra
Vertebral canal	Spinal Canal
Vertebral foramen	Cervical Vertebra
Vertebral foramen	Lumbar Vertebra
Vertebral foramen	Thoracic Vertebra
Vertebral lamina	Cervical Vertebra
Vertebral lamina	Lumbar Vertebra
Vertebral lamina	Thoracic Vertebra
Vertebral pedicle	Cervical Vertebra
Vertebral pedicle	Lumbar Vertebra
Vertebral pedicle	Thoracic Vertebra
Vesical vein	Hypogastric Vein, Right
Vesical vein	Hypogastric Vein, Left
Vestibular (Scarpa's) ganglion	Acoustic Nerve
Vestibular nerve	Acoustic Nerve
Vestibulocochlear nerve (syn)	Acoustic Nerve
Virchow's (supraclavicular) lymph node	Lymphatic, Left Neck
Virchow's (supraclavicular) lymph node	Lymphatic, Right Neck
Vitreous body (syn)	Vitreous, Left
Vitreous body (syn)	Vitreous, Right
Vocal fold (syn)	Vocal Cord, Right
Vocal fold (syn)	Vocal Cord, Left
Volar (palmar) metacarpal vein	Hand Vein, Left
Volar (palmar) digital vein	Hand Vein, Left
Volar (palmar) metacarpal vein	Hand Vein, Right
Volar (palmar) digital vein	Hand Vein, Right
Vomer	Nasal Bone
Vomer	Nasal Septum
Xiphoid process	Sternum
Zonule of Zinn	Lens, Left
Zonule of Zinn	Lens, Right
Zygomatic process of frontal bone	Frontal Bone, Right
Zygomatic process of frontal bone	Frontal Bone, Left

ICD-10 PROCEDURE CODING SYSTEM
MEDICAL/SURGICAL SECTION
BODY PART KEY BY ANATOMICAL TERM

Anatomical Term	PCS Description
Zygomatic process of temporal bone	Temporal Bone, Right
Zygomatic process of temporal bone	Temporal Bone, Left
Zygomaticus muscle	Facial Muscle

Appendix B

(Note: The Root Operation Tables listed in Appendix B contain the same information regarding Root Operations as presented in Appendix A of the 2011 ICD-10-PCS Reference Manual but are presented in a different format.)

Root Operations in the Medical and Surgical Section

Medical and Surgical Section Root Operation Groups

Root Operation	Objective of Procedure	Site of Procedure	Example
Root operations that take out some/all of a body part			
Excision	Cutting out/off without replacement	Some of a body part	Breast lumpectomy
Resection	Cutting out/off without replacement	All of a body part	Total mastectomy
Detachment	Cutting out/off without replacement	Extremity only, any level	Amputation above elbow
Destruction	Eradicating without replacement	Some/all of a body part	Fulguration of endometrium
Extraction	Pulling out or off without replacement	Some/all of a body part	Suction D&C
Root operations that take out solids/fluids/gases from a body part			
Drainage	Taking/letting out fluids/gases	Within a body part	Incision and drainage
Extirpation	Taking/cutting out solid matter	Within a body part	Thrombectomy
Fragmen-tation	Breaking solid matter into pieces	Within a body part	Lithotripsy
Root operations involving cutting or separation only			
Division	Cutting into/separating a body part	Within a body part	Neurotomy
Release	Freeing a body part from constraint	Around a body part	Adhesiolysis
Root operations that put in/put back or move some/all of a body part			
Transplan-tation	Putting in a living body part from a person/animal	Some/all of a body part	Kidney transplant
Reattach-ment	Putting back a detached body part	Some/all of a body part	Reattach severed finger
Transfer	Moving, to function for a similar body part	Some/all of a body part	Skin transfer flap
Reposition	Moving, to normal or other suitable location	Some/all of a body part	Move undescended testicle

Root operations that alter the diameter/route of a tubular body part			
Restriction	Partially closing orifice/lumen	Tubular body part	Gastroesophageal fundoplication
Occlusion	Completely closing orifice/lumen	Tubular body part	Fallopian tube ligation
Dilation	Expanding orifice/lumen	Tubular body part	Percutaneous transluminal coronary angioplasty (PTCA)
Bypass	Altering route of passage	Tubular body part	Coronary artery bypass graft (CABG)
Root operations that always involve a device			
Insertion	Putting in non-biological device	In/on a body part	Central line insertion
Replace-ment	Putting in device that replaces a body part	Some/all of a body part	Total hip replacement
Supple-ment	Putting in device that reinforces or augments a body part	In/on a body part	Abdominal wall herniorrhaphy using mesh
Change	Exchanging device w/out cutting/ puncturing	In/on a body part	Drainage tube change
Removal	Taking out device	In/on a body part	Central line removal
Revision	Correcting a malfunctioning/displaced device	In/on a body part	Revision of pacemaker insertion
Root operations involving examination only			
Inspection	Visual/manual exploration	Some/all of a body part	Diagnostic cystoscopy
Map	Locating electrical impulses/functional areas	Brain/cardiac conduction mechanism	Cardiac electrophysiological study
Root operations that include other repairs			
Repair	Restoring body part to its normal structure	Some/all of a body part	Suture laceration
Control	Stopping/attempting to stop postprocedural bleed	Anatomical region	Post-prostatectomy bleeding
Root operations that include other objectives			
Fusion	Rendering joint immobile	Joint	Spinal fusion
Alteration	Modifying body part for cosmetic purposes without affecting function	Some/all of a body part	Face lift
Creation	Making new structure for sex change operation	Perineum	Artificial vagina/penis

Root Operations in the Medical and Surgical Section in Alphabetical Order

Alteration 0	Definition	Modifying the natural anatomic structure of a body part without affecting the function of the body part
	Explanation	Principal purpose is to improve appearance
	Examples	Face lift, breast augmentation
Bypass 1	Definition	Altering the route of passage of the contents of a tubular body part
	Explanation	Rerouting contents around an area of a body part to another distal (downstream) area in the normal route; rerouting the contents to another different but similar route and body part; or to an abnormal route and another dissimilar body part. It includes one or more concurrent anastomoses with or without the use of a device such as autografts, tissue substitutes and synthetic substitutes
	Examples	Coronary artery bypass graft (CABG), colostomy formation
Change 2	Definition	Taking out or off a device from a body part and putting back an identical or similar device in or on the same body part without cutting or puncturing the skin or a mucous membrane
	Explanation	All Change procedures are coded using the approach External
	Examples	Urinary catheter change, gastrostomy tube change, drainage tube change
Control 3	Definition	Stopping, or attempting to stop, postprocedural bleeding
	Explanation	The site of the bleeding is coded as an anatomical region and not to a specific body part
	Examples	Control of post-prostatectomy hemorrhage, control of post-tonsillectomy hemorrhage
Creation 4	Definition	Making a new genital structure that does not take over the function of a body part
	Explanation	Used only for sex change operations
	Examples	Creation of vagina in a male, creation of penis in a female
Destruction 5	Definition	Physical eradication of all or a portion of a body part by the direct use of energy, force or a destructive agent
	Explanation	None of the body part is physically taken out
	Examples	Fulguration of rectal polyp, cautery of skin lesion, fulguration of endometrium
Detachment 6	Definition	Cutting off all or part of the upper or lower extremities
	Explanation	The body part value is the site of the detachment, with a qualifier if applicable to further specify the level where the extremity was detached
	Examples	Below knee amputation, disarticulation of shoulder, amputation above elbow

Dilation 7	Definition	Expanding an orifice or the lumen of a tubular body part
	Explanation	The orifice can be a natural orifice or an artificially created orifice. Accomplished by stretching a tubular body part using intraluminal pressure or by cutting part of the orifice or wall of the tubular body part
	Examples	Percutaneous transluminal angioplasty, pyloromyotomy, percutaneous transluminal coronary angioplasty (PTCA)
Division 8	Definition	Cutting into a body part without draining fluids and/or gases from the body part in order to separate or transect a body part
	Explanation	All or a portion of the body part is separated into two or more portions
	Examples	Spinal cordotomy, osteotomy, neurotomy
Drainage 9	Definition	Taking or letting out fluids and/or gases from a body part
	Explanation	The qualifier **Diagnostic** is used to identify drainage procedures that are biopsies
	Examples	Thoracentesis, incision and drainage
Excision B	Definition	Cutting out or off, without replacement, a portion of a body part
	Explanation	The qualifier **Diagnostic** is used to identify excision procedures that are biopsies
	Examples	Partial nephrectomy, liver biopsy, breast lumpectomy
Extirpation C	Definition	Taking or cutting out solid matter from a body part
	Explanation	The solid matter may be an abnormal byproduct of a biological function or a foreign body; it may be embedded in a body part, or in the lumen of a tubular body part. The solid matter may or may not have been previously broken into pieces.
	Examples	Thrombectomy, choledocholithotomy, excision foreign body
Extraction D	Definition	Pulling or stripping out or off all or a portion of a body part by the use of force
	Explanation	The qualifier **Diagnostic** is used to identify extraction procedures that are biopsies
	Examples	Dilation and curettage, vein stripping, suction D&C, D&C7
Fragmen- tation F	Definition	Breaking solid matter in a body part into pieces
	Explanation	The solid matter may be an abnormal byproduct of a biological function or a foreign body. Physical force (e.g., manual, ultrasonic) applied directly or indirectly through intervening body parts is used to break the solid matter into pieces. The pieces of solid matter are not taken out, but are eliminated or absorbed through normal biological functions
	Examples	Extracorporeal shockwave lithotripsy, transurethral lithotripsy

Fusion G	Definition	Joining together portions of an articular body part rendering the articular body part immobile
	Explanation	The body part is joined together by fixation device, bone graft, or other means
	Examples	Spinal fusion, ankle arthrodesis
Insertion H	Definition	Putting in a non-biological appliance that monitors, assists, performs or prevents a physiological function but does not physically take the place of a body part
	Explanation	N/A
	Examples	Insertion of radioactive implant, insertion of central venous catheter
Inspection J	Definition	Visually and/or manually exploring a body part
	Explanation	Visual exploration may be performed with or without optical instrumentation. Manual exploration may be performed directly or through intervening body layers
	Examples	Diagnostic arthroscopy, exploratory laparotomy, diagnostic cystoscopy
Map K	Definition	Locating the route of passage of electrical impulses and/or locating functional areas in a body part
	Explanation	Applicable only to the cardiac conduction mechanism and the central nervous system
	Examples	Cardiac mapping, cortical mapping, cardiac electrophysiological study
Occlusion L	Definition	Completely closing an orifice or the lumen of a tubular body part
	Explanation	The orifice can be a natural orifice or an artificially created orifice
	Examples	Fallopian tube ligation, ligation of inferior vena cava
Reattach- ment M	Definition	Putting back in or on all or a portion of a separated body part to its normal location or other suitable location
	Explanation	Vascular circulation and nervous pathways may or may not be reestablished
	Examples	Reattachment of hand, reattachment of avulsed kidney, reattachment of finger
Release N	Definition	Freeing a body part from an abnormal physical constraint
	Explanation	Some of the restraining tissue may be taken out but none of the body part is taken out
	Examples	Adhesiolysis, carpal tunnel release

Removal P	Definition	Taking out or off a device from a body part
	Explanation	If the device is taken out and a similar device is put in without cutting or puncturing the skin or mucous membrane, the procedure is coded to the root operation Change. Otherwise, the procedure for taking out the device is coded to the root operation Removal and the procedure for putting in the new device is coded to the root operation performed.
	Examples	Drainage tube removal, cardiac pacemaker removal, central line removal
Repair Q	Definition	Restoring, to the extent possible, a body part to its normal anatomic structure and function
	Explanation	Used only when the method to accomplish the repair is not one of the other root operations
	Examples	Herniorrhaphy, suture of laceration
Replacement R	Definition	Putting in or on biological or synthetic material that physically takes the place and/or function of all or a portion of a body part
	Explanation	The biological material is non-living, or the biological material is living and from the same individual. The body part may have been previously taken out, previously replaced, or may be taken out concomitantly with the Replacement procedure. **If the body part has been previously replaced, a separate Removal procedure is coded for taking out the device used in the previous replacement.**
	Examples	Total hip replacement, bone graft, free skin graft
Reposition S	Definition	Moving to its normal location or other suitable location all or a portion of a body part
	Explanation	The body part is moved to a new location from an abnormal location, or from a normal location where it is not functioning correctly. The body part may or may not be cut out or off to be moved to the new location.
	Examples	Reposition of undescended testicle, fracture reduction
Resection T	Definition	Cutting out or off, without replacement, all of a body part
	Explanation	N/A
	Examples	Total nephrectomy, total lobectomy of lung, total mastectomy
Restriction V	Definition	Partially closing an orifice or the lumen of a tubular body part
	Explanation	The orifice can be a natural orifice or an artificially created orifice
	Examples	Esophagogastric fundoplication, cervical cerclage

Revision W	Definition	Correcting, to the extent possible, a malfunctioning or displaced device
	Explanation	Revision can include correcting a malfunctioning or displaced device by taking out or putting in components of the device such as a screw or pin
	Examples	Adjustment of pacemaker lead, adjustment of hip prosthesis, revision of pacemaker insertion
Supplement U	Definition	Putting in or on biologic or synthetic material that physically reinforces and/or augments the function of a portion of a body part
	Explanation	The biological material is non-living, or the biological material is living and from the same individual. The body part may have been previously replaced. If the body part has been previously replaced, the Supplement procedure is performed to physically reinforce and/or augment the function of the replaced body part.
	Examples	Herniorrhaphy using mesh, free nerve graft, mitral valve ring annuloplasty, put a new acetabular liner in a previous hip replacement, abdominal wall herniorrhaphy using mesh
Transfer X	Definition	Moving, without taking out, all or a portion of a body part to another location to take over the function of all or a portion of a body part
	Explanation	The body part transferred remains connected to its vascular and nervous supply
	Examples	Tendon transfer, skin pedicle flap transfer, skin transfer flap
Transplan- tation Y	Definition	Putting in or on all or a portion of a living body part taken from another individual or animal to physically take the place and/or function of all or a portion of a similar body part
	Explanation	The native body part may or may not be taken out, and the transplanted body part may take over all or a portion of its function
	Examples	Kidney transplant, heart transplant

Appendix C

(Note: The Approach Table listed in Appendix C contains the same information regarding Approaches as presented in Appendix A of the 2011 ICD-10-PCS Reference Manual but is presented in a different format.)

ICD-10-PCS Approaches

Value	Approach	Definition	Examples
0	**Open**	Cutting through the skin or mucous membrane and any other body layers necessary to expose the site of the procedure	Open CABG Open endarterectomy Open resection cecum Abdominal hysterectomy
3	**Percutaneous**	Entry, by puncture or minor incision, of instrumentation through the skin or mucous membrane and any other body layers necessary to reach the site of the procedure	Percutaneous needle core biopsy of kidney Liposuction Percutaneous drainage of ascites Needle biopsy of liver
4	**Percutaneous Endoscopic**	Entry, by puncture or minor incision, of instrumentation through the skin or mucous membrane and any other body layers necessary to reach and visualize the site of the procedure	Laparoscopic cholecystectomy Laparoscopy with destruction of endometriosis Endoscopic drainage of sinus Arthroscopy
7	**Via Natural or Artificial Opening**	Entry of instrumentation through a natural or artificial external opening to reach the site of the procedure	Foley catheter placement Transvaginal intraluminal cervical cerclage Digital rectal exam Endotracheal intubation
8	**Via Natural or Artificial Opening Endoscopic**	Entry of instrumentation through a natural or artificial external opening to reach and visualize the site of the procedure	Transurethral cystoscopy with removal of bladder stone Endoscopic ERCP Hysteroscopy EGD Colonoscopy
F	**Via Natural or Artificial Opening with Percutaneous Endoscopic Assistance**	Entry of instrumentation through a natural or artificial external opening and entry, by puncture or minor incision, of instrumentation through the skin or mucous membrane and any other body layers necessary to aid in the performance of the procedure	Laparoscopic-assisted vaginal hysterectomy
X	**External**	Procedures performed directly on the skin or mucous membrane and procedures performed indirectly by the application of external force through the skin or mucous membrane	Resection of tonsils Closed reduction of fracture Excision of skin lesion Cautery nosebleed

AHIMA ICD-10 Products

Available at www.ahimastore.org

Books from AHIMA Press

- *Implementing ICD-10-CM/PCS for Hospitals* (AC201009)
- *Pocket Guide of ICD-10-CM and ICD-10-PCS* (AC203010)
- *ICD-10-CM and ICD-10-PCS Preview*, Second Edition (AC206009)
- *ICD-10-CM and ICD-10-PCS Preview Exercises*, Second Edition (AC216011)
- *ICD-10-CM Coder Training Manual 2011* (AC206811)
- *ICD-10-PCS Coder Training Manual 2011* (AC207811)
- *Transitioning to ICD-10-CM/PCS: The Essential Guide to General Equivalence Mappings (GEMs)* (AC202810)
- *Root Operations: Key to Procedure Coding in ICD-10-PCS (*AC211010)

AHIMA Online Education

- *ICD-10-CM Overview: Deciphering the Code Course*
- *ICD-10-PCS Overview: Deciphering the Code Course*
- *Coding Proficiency Assessments*
  - *ICD-10-CM Coding Assessment*
  - *ICD-10-PCS Coding Assessment*
  - *ICD-10 A&P System Coding Assessments*
- *ICD-10 Overview: Mortality Reporting Course*
- *ICD-10-CM/PCS: Fundamentals of General Equivalence Mapping (GEMs) Course*
- *Documentation Improvement in Preparing for ICD-10-CM/PCS Course*

AHIMA Meetings (Check AHIMA.org for dates)

- Annual ICD-10 Summit
- Academy for ICD-10-CM/PCS Trainers (nationwide, near you)
- Private Academies (Contact AHIMA Business Development Office)
- AHIMA Annual Convention and Exhibits

AHIMA Audio Seminars and Webinars

- Check AHIMA.org for dates and topics

Codebooks from Ingenix

- *ICD-10-CM: The Complete Official Draft Code Set (2011) (VC209111)*
- *ICD-10-PCS: The Complete Official Draft Code Set (2011) (VC209211)*
- *ICD-10-CM Mappings (VC201911)*